WALL PILATES WORKOUT FOR WOMEN OVER 40

6 Minutes Daily Simple Low Impact Exercise for Weight loss, improved cardiovascular function, Enhanced posture, Independence and balance

Novella D. Thompson

TABLE OF CONTENT

INTRODUCTION

Tracy was caught up in the rush and bustle of modern life when she encountered an all-too-familiar adversary: chronic pain and suffering. Each morning appeared to bring a new agony, a reminder of the toll that years of neglect had placed on her body.

Waist discomfort became a frequent companion, its sharp twinges providing an unwanted soundtrack to her everyday activities. Tracy's once-active lifestyle had given way to a sedentary one, accompanied by constant joint discomfort, leaving her feeling trapped and despondent.

Despite her best attempts to ease the agony in different ways, Tracy faced an uphill struggle. Her previous attempts at traditional procedures only gave brief comfort, prompting her to seek a more long-term

remedy. Tracy came upon a book titled "
Wall Pilates Workout for Women Over 40" at
a particularly depressing period.

Tracy was hooked as she read the book's
promise of newfound vigor and power.
Pilates concepts spoke to her deeply,
providing a comprehensive approach to
wellbeing that appeared to be tailored to her
specific requirements.

 Tracy, determined to restore her health and
vigor, went on a path of self-discovery,
devoting herself completely to the book's
lessons.

Tracy, armed with newfound information and
a renewed sense of purpose, began
applying Pilates movements at home, taking
modest but methodical steps toward
regaining her health.

With each gentle exercise, she felt the
tightness in her muscles melt away, leaving

behind a renewed sensation of power and flexibility. Tracy's metamorphosis grew more visible as the days passed and the weeks evolved into months.

Gone were the days of waist pain and stiffness; instead, a woman was empowered by her endurance and resolve. Tracy embraced her newfound life with boundless zest, grabbing every opportunity to enjoy it to the utmost. Tracy's world grew in ways she never expected, from discovering new activities to reconnecting with old ones.

Tracy is now a living example of Pilates' transformational potential and the indomitable human spirit. Through effort and determination, she not only overcame her physical illnesses, but also emerged stronger and more vibrant than before. Tracy reflects on her path and is appreciative for the part Pilates played in her life, as well as the second opportunity it provided.

Chapter 1: The Principles of Pilates

Pilates is a type of exercise that aims to strengthen the body, increase flexibility, and improve overall physical and mental health. Pilates, which was developed by Joseph Pilates in the early twentieth century, has grown in popularity across the world due to its efficacy in increasing core strength, balance, and coordination.

Several ideas underpin Pilate's practice, guiding its philosophy and approach. Understanding these concepts is critical for maximizing the advantages of Pilates training. Here, we look at the essential concepts of Pilates, describing each one succinctly and directly.

1. *Focus:* In Pilates, focus is essential. Each exercise takes complete concentration and mindfulness. By focusing on the present moment and doing each exercise precisely, practitioners may strengthen their mind-body connection, increase body awareness, and improve overall movement efficiency.

2. *Control:* Pilates emphasizes control to promote safe and effective movement patterns. Rather than depending on momentum or physical force, practitioners learn to move with precision and elegance, utilizing their muscles under control. This helps to avoid injuries, encourages good alignment, and optimizes the benefits of each activity.

3. *Centering:* Central to Pilates is the notion of centering, which focuses on the core muscles, sometimes known as the "powerhouse." By activating the muscles of the belly, lower back, hips, and buttocks, practitioners stabilize the body and provide a solid foundation for movement. Centering strengthens the core while also improving posture and general body alignment.

4. Breathing: Pilates focuses on a certain breathing rhythm that coincides with movement. Practitioners are urged to breathe deeply and regularly, utilizing the diaphragm to expand the lungs and contract the deep abdominal muscles.

Proper breathing oxygenates the blood, promotes relaxation, and increases the flow of energy throughout the body, allowing for smoother, more fluid movement.

5. Precision: Precision is essential in Pilates. Each movement is executed with painstaking attention to detail, emphasizing perfect alignment, form, and technique. By improving movement patterns and perfecting accuracy, practitioners may more efficiently target particular muscle groups, obtain optimal outcomes, and reduce the chance of injury.

6. *Flow:* Pilates movements are meant to transition smoothly from one to the next, resulting in a continuous and fluid movement experience.

Flowing movement sequences boost circulation flexibility, and produce a sense of calm and well-being. Throughout their Pilates practice, practitioners seek to maintain a fluid and rhythmic flow, bringing the mind, body, and breath together in harmony.

7. *Integration:* Pilates strives to integrate the entire body rather than isolating certain muscles or bodily sections. Practitioners gain functional strength, coordination, and balance through integrated movement patterns, which they then use for everyday tasks and sports performance. Integration develops mental and physical oneness, fostering overall health and well-being.

By applying these ideas into our Pilates practice, you may dramatically improve your physical strength, flexibility, and overall health.

Whether you're a novice or a seasoned practitioner, adopting the concepts of attention, control, centering, breathing, accuracy, flow, and integration will help you comprehend Pilates and maximize its advantages. Maintain mindfulness and attention while enjoying the path of self-discovery and self-improvement that Pilates provides.

Understanding the Basics

Pilates, a low-impact workout program that focuses on strength, flexibility, and endurance, has grown in popularity among women over 40 owing to its potential to enhance posture, core strength, and overall fitness levels.

Wall Pilates is a variant of classic Pilates that uses a wall as a prop to improve stability, support, and alignment during exercises. Here's a detailed look at the fundamentals of Wall Pilates routines designed for ladies over 40:

1. Foundation and Alignment: Wall Pilates focuses on appropriate alignment and posture to improve performance and prevent injury. Women over 40 frequently encounter changes in their bodies, such as reduced bone density and muscle mass, making proper alignment critical for safety and efficacy.

2. *Core Strengthening:* As women age, core strength becomes increasingly important for maintaining stability, balance, and functional mobility. Wall Pilates works the deep core muscles, especially the transverse abdominis and pelvic floor, to strengthen and stabilize the spine.

3. *Improved Flexibility and Mobility:* To prevent a decrease with age, Wall Pilates routines should include stretching and mobility movements. The wall acts as a guide for appropriate alignment during stretches, resulting in increased flexibility and range of motion.

4. *Balance and Stability:* Women over 40 may struggle with balance and stability owing to age-related changes in proprioception and muscular strength. Wall Pilates exercises improve balance and stability by using the wall as support while completing movements that require coordination and control.

5. *Mind-Body Connection:* Pilates encourages attention and awareness of movement patterns. Wall Pilates routines urge women over 40 to focus on breath control, attention, and accuracy to improve exercise efficacy and induce relaxation.

6. *Progression and Modification:* Wall Pilates exercises may be tailored to different fitness levels and skills. Women over the age of 40 can make modest improvements by by increasing the intensity or duration of their workouts while listening to the bodies body and avoiding overtraining.

7. *Consistency and Patience:* Effective Wall Pilates requires consistency and patience, just like any other workout. Women over the age of 40 should commit to regular practice while realizing that improvement takes time and varies by person.

Wall Pilates workouts provide various advantages to women over 40, including increased posture, core strength, flexibility, balance, and stability. Women may improve their general health and well-being by grasping the fundamentals and applying them to their daily routines with this simple and effective workout strategy.

Benefits of Wall Pilates for Women Over 40

Wall Pilates, a creative version of conventional Pilates movements, provides several benefits, particularly for women over 40. As women age, maintaining flexibility, strength, and general well-being becomes increasingly vital.

Wall Pilates meets these requirements swiftly and effectively, offering a low-impact but extremely effective workout. Let's look at the entire benefits of Wall Pilates for ladies over 40.

Improved Posture: As we age, our posture deteriorates owing to a variety of causes such as sedentary lives and weakened muscles. Wall Pilates emphasizes core strength and alignment, which aids in correcting bad posture patterns. Women over 40 may improve their posture significantly by using their core muscles and aligning themselves properly against the wall, resulting in less back discomfort and more confidence.

Enhanced Flexibility: Flexibility is essential for preserving mobility and avoiding injuries as we age. Wall Pilates combines stretching movements that target muscles across the body, increasing flexibility and joint mobility.

This is especially advantageous for women over 40 since it counteracts the natural loss of flexibility that comes with aging, allowing them to move more freely and pleasantly in their regular activities.

Increased Strength: As women age, building and maintaining muscle strength becomes increasingly essential since it can help prevent age-related muscle loss (sarcopenia) and preserve bone density.

Wall Pilates strengthens muscles by using bodyweight resistance exercises and the wall as support, notably in the core, arms, legs, and back. This helps women over 40 retain functional strength for everyday tasks while also lowering the risk of falls and accidents.

Joint Health: Women over the age of 40 frequently complain about joint pain and stiffness, particularly if they have arthritis. Wall Pilates is a mild but efficient approach to promote joint health by lubricating the joints with regulated motions while improving blood flow to the surrounding tissues. Wall Pilates' low-impact nature makes it ideal for anyone with joint concerns, letting them build muscles without increasing pain or discomfort.

Stress Relief: As women balance several obligations and face life's problems, stress management becomes increasingly crucial. Wall Pilates combines focused breathing methods with fluid movements to promote relaxation and stress alleviation. Women over 40 who focus on the present moment and connect with their bodies can reduce stress, improve mental clarity, and improve their general well-being.

Core Stability: Core strength is critical for maintaining balance, stability, and good alignment, particularly as women age. Wall Pilates stresses core activation in all of its exercises, assisting women over 40 in developing a strong and stable core. This not only improves posture and lowers the chance of injury, but it also boosts performance in other physical activities and sports.

Mind-Body Connection: Wall Pilates promotes a strong connection between the mind and body, resulting in increased body awareness and mindfulness. Women over 40 who practice mindful movement and focus on good alignment can enhance their coordination, balance, and proprioception. This increased awareness translates into daily life, allowing people to move more effectively and with better ease.

Wall Pilates provides several benefits for women over 40, addressing their specific requirements while also boosting overall health and well-being.

From better posture and flexibility to greater strength and joint health, this novel type of training offers a full workout that can help women stay active, healthy, and vibrant as they become older.

Women over 40 who incorporate Wall Pilates into their training program will reap several physical and emotional advantages that will help them on their path to maximum health and vitality.

Safety Precautions and Considerations

Wall Pilates routines have various advantages for women over 40, including increased strength, flexibility, and posture. However, prioritizing safety is critical for avoiding injuries and increasing the efficacy of your exercise. Keep in mind the following complete safety measures and considerations:

Consultation with a Healthcare Professional: Before beginning any new fitness regimen, particularly if you are over 40, you should consult with your healthcare professional. They may evaluate your specific health situation and make tailored suggestions.

Warm-up and Cool-down: Start each training session with a mild warm-up to prepare your muscles and joints for movement. Similarly, finish with a cool-down session to assist your body return to a resting condition and lessen the likelihood of muscular discomfort.

Mindful Movement: Throughout your Wall Pilates exercise, focus on mindful movement and good technique. Maintain proper body posture and prevent overexertion or quick, jerky movements that may strain muscles or joints.

Start Slowly and Progress progressively: If you're new to Pilates or haven't exercised in a while, begin with simple exercises and progressively increase the intensity and complexity as your strength and competence improve.

Listen to your body. Respect your body's limitations and don't push through pain or discomfort. If you encounter any odd or chronic pain while exercising, stop immediately and see a medical practitioner.

Use Proper Equipment: Make sure you have a strong and solid wall surface for your Pilates routines. Purchase high-quality equipment, such as a Pilates mat and any other props or accessories advised for your program.

keep Hydrated: Drink lots of water before, during, and after your workouts to keep hydrated and promote proper muscle function.

Modify as Needed: Don't be afraid to change workouts to meet your own requirements and talents. Use props or changes to make motions more accessible or difficult as needed.

Breathing Awareness: Keep your breath steady and regulated throughout your workouts. Proper breathing can help you perform better, get more oxygen into your muscles, and relax.

Regular Rest and Recovery: Include rest days in your workout regimen to give your body time to heal and repair. Adequate rest is critical for avoiding burnout and lowering the likelihood of overuse problems.

Women over 40 may reap the advantages of Wall Pilates sessions while lowering their chance of injury and improving their general well-being by following these safety measures and considerations.

Chapter 2: Setting Up Your Space

Setting up your area for wall pilates exercises, especially for women over 40, necessitates careful planning to guarantee safety, comfort, and efficacy. Here's a complete guide to help you establish a perfect configuration:

Choose the Right Location: Choose a location in your house with ample space to roam about. Consider a calm environment where you can concentrate without distractions.

Clear the Area: Remove any furniture or obstructions that may be impeding your movements. Clearing the area provides a safe atmosphere for performing workouts without the chance of colliding with things.

Prepare the Wall: Make sure the wall you'll be utilizing is clean and clear of any sharp items or uneven surfaces that might cause harm. A smooth, level wall surface is essential for maintaining stability when exercising.

Gather Required Equipment: Gather your pilates mat, resistance bands, and any other equipment you will be utilizing during the exercises. Having everything within reach saves time and helps you stay focused on the workouts.

Consider Lighting: Proper lighting is necessary for safety and visibility. Choose a well-lit place or add extra lighting to ensure you can see well.

Improve Ventilation: Proper airflow in your training area helps to control temperature and keeps you comfortable while exercising. Maintain appropriate ventilation by opening windows or using fans.

Set a supportive atmosphere for your workout by playing peaceful music or using aromatherapy. Creating a peaceful environment might improve your attention and motivation.

Check for Safety risks: Examine the area for any possible risks, such as loose carpets or slick flooring. Addressing these issues ahead of time minimizes the likelihood of injury throughout your exercises.

Adjust for Accessibility: If you have mobility issues or physical restrictions, make accommodations to meet your requirements. Use props or adjust exercises as needed to ensure accessibility and safety.

Maintain Organization: Keep your workout area neat and clutter-free to reduce distractions and streamline your routines.

Use storage options to keep equipment neatly kept while not in use.

By following these measures, you may create an ideal setting for wall pilates exercises for women over 40. Prioritizing safety, comfort, and accessibility leads to a great workout experience that helps you achieve your health and wellness objectives.

Creating a Pilates-Friendly Environment

Proper Equipment: Purchase high-quality Pilates mats, resistance bands, stability balls, and Pilates-specific props. For wall Pilates, use robust wall-mounted bars or equipment to provide support and stability.

Comfortable Space: Set aside a clean, roomy place with ample ventilation and natural light to practice Pilates movements. A clutter-free environment decreases distractions and the danger of damage.

Prioritize safety by keeping all equipment properly maintained and in good shape. Install non slip flooring to avoid injuries, particularly during dynamic motions. To avoid pain and injury, provide appropriate cushioning for sensitive regions such as the knees and elbows.

Temperature Control: Keep the room at a reasonable temperature for exercise, usually between 68 and 72 degrees Fahrenheit (20-22 degrees Celsius). This helps to minimize overheating and maintains peak performance throughout exercises.

Ambiance: Use soft lighting, soothing music, and a few distractions to create a serene environment. Encourage participants to concentrate on their breathing and movements, so promoting awareness and relaxation.

Customization Options: Meet individual requirements and preferences by providing a choice of adaptations and progressions for different fitness levels and talents. Encourage participants to listen to their bodies and make necessary modifications to guarantee a safe and productive workout.

Hire certified Pilates teachers who have experience dealing with women over 40 and customizing routines to different fitness levels and health issues. Clear, succinct cueing helps participants comprehend and execute motions correctly, lowering their risk of injury.

Community Support: Create a helpful and inclusive environment in which participants feel encouraged and inspired to attain their fitness objectives. Create chances for social engagement and networking, such as post-workout chats or gatherings.

Regular Maintenance: Check the equipment to verify it is working and safe. Cleaning and sanitizing equipment after each use promotes hygiene and prevents germ transmission.

Comments Mechanism: Create open communication routes for participants to share comments and recommendations for enhancing the Pilates experience. Actively listen to their feedback and make any required improvements to improve their overall experience.

By applying these ideas, you may establish a Pilates-friendly atmosphere that caters to the specific requirements of women over 40 who participate in wall Pilates exercises, improving their health, well-being, and pleasure of the exercise.

Choosing the Right Wall

When it comes to wall Pilates workouts for women over 40, selecting the appropriate wall is critical for safety, comfort, and efficacy. Here's a detailed guide on choosing the ideal wall for your Pilates routine:

Stability and Support: Choose a wall that is solid and stable. It should be able to sustain your body weight without wobbling or trembling, particularly during activities that require leaning or pressing on it.

Smooth Surface: Choose a wall with a smooth surface to avoid pain or abrasions during activities that involve direct contact with the wall, such as wall sits or push-ups.

Ample room: Make sure the wall has adequate room around it to allow for the complete range of motion. You should be able to travel freely, with no impediments or barriers close.

Cleanliness: Prioritize cleanliness by choosing a clean wall that is free of dirt, dust, and other pollutants. This is especially critical if you will be pressing your hands or torso against the wall during activities.

Accessibility: Select a wall that is conveniently accessible inside your training area. It should be easy to access and perfectly positioned to promote good alignment and posture during activity.

Visual Appeal: While not required for optimal workout results, choosing a visually appealing wall might improve your whole exercise experience. Consider color, texture, and aesthetics while designing a comfortable atmosphere for your Pilates practice.

Safety precautions: Look for any potential risks or protrusions on the wall's surface that might cause a risk during exercise. Smooth edges and rounded corners are preferable over sharp or jagged surfaces.

Versatility: Choose a wall that allows you to execute different sorts of activities. Look for features like adjustable bars, hooks, or connection points that allow you to incorporate a wide range of Pilates routines and equipment into your workouts.

Following these rules will ensure that you select the appropriate wall for your Pilates practices as a woman over 40.

Consider stability, comfort, and safety to get the most out of your workout and avoid injuries. With the ideal wall as your base, you may have a rewarding and productive Pilates practice for years to come.

Essential Equipment and Props

Wall Pilates routines are an excellent approach for women over 40 to increase their strength, flexibility, and general fitness levels.

Incorporating necessary equipment and props into these workouts can increase efficacy and give extra assistance. Here's a detailed list of the needed equipment and props for Wall Pilates workouts:

Pilates Mat: While Wall Pilates relies heavily on the wall for support and resistance, a comfortable Pilates mat is vital for cushioning and support during floor exercises and stretches. Look for a high-quality mat with enough thickness and grip to prevent slippage.

Resistance bands are excellent instruments for increasing the intensity of Wall Pilates routines. They offer resistance throughout the activity, so efficiently strengthening and toning the muscles. Select bands with variable degrees of resistance to meet different activities and fitness levels.

Pilates balls, also known as stability balls, bring difficulty and instability to workouts, activating core muscles and increasing balance. It may be used for workouts against the wall or on the mat, providing support for a variety of motions and stretching.

Yoga Blocks: Yoga blocks can be useful for adjusting exercises and giving additional support, particularly for women over 40 who may require extra help with balance or flexibility. They can be used to elevate the hands or feet while performing particular exercises, providing for appropriate alignment and range of movement.

Small Pilates Props: Hand weights, ankle weights, and foam rollers can be used in Wall Pilates sessions to target particular muscle regions while also increasing general strength and stability.

Hand weights can provide resistance to arm workouts, while ankle weights can increase the difficulty of leg activities. Foam rollers are great for reducing tension and increasing flexibility.

A wall-mounted barre is a useful tool for ladies who want to incorporate ballet-inspired routines into their Wall Pilates regimen. It adds stability and support to movements like pliés, relevés, and leg lifts, which assist in developing and toning the lower body.

Women over 40 who invest in these crucial tools and props may improve their Wall Pilates sessions, resulting in better strength, flexibility, and general well-being. Whether you're a novice or a seasoned pro, including these tools in your regimen will improve the efficacy and enjoyment of your exercises.

Tips for Proper Alignment and Posture

Proper alignment and posture are critical to general health and well-being, particularly as we age. Women over 40 can benefit from adopting mindful alignment methods into their training regimens, especially with Wall Pilates programs.

Here are some detailed and straightforward recommendations for maintaining appropriate alignment and posture throughout Wall Pilates exercises:

Mindful Awareness: Begin each practice by focusing on your body's alignment. Before beginning your workout, take a minute to check your posture and make any required corrections.

Maintain a neutral spine during the workouts. This involves preserving the natural curvature of the spine, with no undue arching or rounding of the back.

Shoulder Alignment: Keep your shoulders relaxed and down, away from your ears. Avoid hunching forward or tensing your shoulders when moving. Imagine moving your shoulder blades down your back to promote appropriate alignment.

Engage Core Muscles: Use your core muscles to stabilize your spine and pelvis. Draw the navel in towards the spine and work the deep abdominal muscles throughout the movements.

Hip Alignment: For stability and balance, align your hips with your shoulders and ankles. Avoid shifting the pelvis too much forward or backward.

Knee Positioning: Keep your knees aligned with your ankles and avoid locking them during exercises. To decrease joint strain, keep your knees slightly bent.

Foot Placement: Ground through all four corners of your feet, distributing weight evenly between the heels and balls. Avoid rolling on the inner or outer margins of your feet.

Breath Awareness: To encourage relaxation and flow, make sure your breath matches your motions. During the preparation phase of each exercise, inhale deeply through the nose, then exhale completely through the mouth as you activate the muscles and do the action.

Use Props for Support: Place props like foam blocks or a stability ball against the wall to give support and help as needed, especially if you have restricted mobility or balance problems.

Listen to your body. Pay attention to any discomfort or strain during the exercises, and adjust or stop any motions that cause pain. Respect your body's limitations and go at your speed.

Including these principles in your Wall Pilates routines will assist women over 40 improve their alignment, posture, and general physical health.

Prioritizing good alignment not only improves the efficacy of your exercises but also lowers the chance of injury and promotes long-term health.

Chapter 3: Foundation Building for Core Strengthening

Core strength is critical for general stability, posture, and movement efficiency, particularly as we age. Women over 40 frequently have reduced muscle mass and bone density, making core strengthening workouts essential for preserving health and mobility.

Foundation building for core strengthening entails a methodical approach to progressively increasing stability and strength in the muscles that support the spine and pelvis. Here's a thorough introduction to basic exercises, with a focus on Wall Pilates Workouts for Women Over 40.

Understanding Core Muscles: Before beginning workouts, it's critical to grasp the core muscles. These include both the superficial abdominals and deeper stabilizing muscles such as the transverse abdominis, pelvic floor, and multifidus.

Starting with Stability: Begin by learning fundamental stability exercises that work the core without causing excessive movement. Wall exercises, such as standing with your back to the wall and executing pelvic tilts or light abdominal compressions, are ideal for this purpose.

Gradual Progression: Slowly increase the complexity and intensity of your exercises. For example, after fundamental stability has been established, go to exercises such as wall squats or leg lifts against the wall, which engage the core dynamically while giving support.

Pilates principles include core strength, stability, and flexibility. Use Pilates principles like breathing, accuracy, control, and fluid movement in your wall exercises. Moves such as wall roll-ups and wall plank variants may efficiently train the core while incorporating Pilates concepts.

Maintaining Proper Alignment: Pay particular attention to your alignment during each exercise. Proper alignment targets the proper muscles while reducing the chance of injury. The wall can provide a tactile signal for alignment, allowing you to maintain good posture and technique.

Consistency and Progress Tracking: Consistency is essential for noticing outcomes. Aim to include core workouts in your regimen at least three to four times each week. Monitor your development by measuring changes in strength, endurance, and posture over time.

Women over 40 can increase stability, lower the chance of injury, and improve their general quality of life by concentrating on foundational strengthening via specific core exercises, notably Wall Pilates Workouts.

Always check with a fitness expert or a healthcare practitioner before starting any new workout routine, especially if you have any pre-existing health issues.

Engaging the Powerhouse

Women over 40 are finding the transforming effects of Wall Pilates exercises as they strive for peak health and fitness. These dynamic workouts not only activate the core muscle but also provide several benefits customized to the demands of this group.

Wall Pilates, a version of classic Pilates, uses the support and resistance of a wall to improve stability, balance, and strength. At their heart, these workouts target the deep abdominal muscles, pelvic floor, and back muscles, also known as the powerhouse.

Women over 40 who use these muscles can improve their posture, relieve back discomfort, and increase their general mobility.

One of the main advantages of Wall Pilates for women over 40 is its low-impact nature. Unlike high-intensity exercises, which can strain joints and aggravate existing ailments, Wall Pilates provides a gentle yet effective technique to build muscles and enhance flexibility while avoiding damage. This makes it an excellent alternative for anyone who has joint concerns or wants to ease into a workout regimen.

Wall Pilates routines are simply adaptable to suit different fitness levels and skills. Whether you're a novice or a seasoned practitioner, the exercises may be adapted to your specific needs, assuring a safe and satisfying experience.

The use of props like stability balls and resistance bands may offer diversity and challenge to exercises, keeping them interesting and effective.

mental well-being is promoted through Wall pilates beyond the physical benefits

The emphasis on breath control and concentration during each practice promotes relaxation and stress alleviation, making it a wonderful antidote to the pressures of daily life.

As women deal with the stresses of job, family, and aging, including these thoughtful techniques into their workout regimen may bring a much-needed feeling of balance and calm.

Wall Pilates routines provide women over 40 with a holistic approach to health and fitness. These exercises enable people to enjoy active, vibrant lives far into their senior years by exercising key muscles, improving posture, and enhancing mental well-being.

Whether you want to reduce pain, increase strength, or just live a better lifestyle, Wall Pilates offers a varied and practical option.

Pelvic Floor Activation Techniques

Pelvic floor activation strategies are vital for women over 40 who participate in Wall Pilates programs. These exercises work the muscles that support the pelvic organs, increasing stability, bladder control, and total core strength. Here's a detailed description of pelvic floor activation techniques designed for ladies over 40 in Wall Pilates workouts:

Deep Breathing: Start by focusing on deep diaphragmatic breathing, which allows the pelvic floor muscles to spontaneously engage and release with each breath. This basic method increases awareness of the pelvic floor and its relationship to the breath.

Kegel exercises consist of tightening and releasing the pelvic floor muscles to strengthen them. Include Kegels in your regimen by pressing the pelvic floor as if to block the flow of pee, holding for a few seconds, and then releasing. Repeat in sets throughout the workout.

Bridge posture Variations: Vary the bridge posture to work the glutes, hamstrings, and pelvic floor muscles at the same time. Lift the hips off the ground, engage the pelvic floor, and then drop with control. This action strengthens the whole pelvic area.

Leg Lifts: Use the pelvic floor to support the pelvis and lower back. Lie on your back, legs stretched or bent, and elevate one leg at a time while keeping the pelvic floor engaged. Alternate legs to cover both sides equally.

Pelvic Tilts: Use pelvic tilts to activate and strengthen your pelvic floor muscles. Lie on your back, legs bent and slowly tilt the pelvis forward and backward while activating the pelvic floor. This activity increases pelvic stability and flexibility.

Wall squats can help strengthen the pelvic floor, thighs, and glutes. Stand with your back to a wall and drop into a squat, activating your pelvic floor as you rise back up. Concentrate on appropriate alignment and precise motions.

Pelvic Clock Visualization: Visualize a clock above your pelvis and move it through the hours by activating your pelvic floor. This visualization approach improves pelvic floor awareness and coordination.

Incorporating pelvic floor activation methods into Wall Pilates routines for women over 40 improves core stability, bladder control, and general pelvic health. Consistency and appropriate form are essential for reaping the advantages of these workouts.

Transverse Abdominis Strengthening

Transverse abdominis (TVA) strengthening is essential, especially for women over 40, since it helps to maintain core stability and supports the spine, improving posture and lowering the chance of injury. Wall Pilates routines are a great way to target and develop your transverse abdominis.

The transverse abdominis is a deep core muscle that helps stabilize the pelvis and spine. Unlike other core muscles, it runs horizontally across the abdomen, functioning as a corset to stabilize and support the whole core.

Core strength is especially crucial for women over 40. Weakness in the transverse abdominis can cause back discomfort, poor posture, and instability, all of which are frequent in older persons. Strengthening this muscle group can help with these ailments and enhance your general quality of life.

Wall Pilates movements provide a unique way to address the transverse abdominis. Individuals who use the wall for support can isolate and work the deep core muscles more efficiently, optimizing benefits while reducing pressure on the lower back.

Key exercises:

Wall Sit with Pelvic Tilt: Stand with your back against the wall and lower yourself into a squat position, holding your knees at 90 degrees. Pull your navel towards your spine to engage your transverse abdominis, then hold for 30-60 seconds.

Wall Plank: Begin in a plank posture with your forearms against the wall and elbows exactly beneath your shoulders. Maintain a straight line from head to heels by using your core muscles, particularly the transverse abdominis, for 30-60 seconds.

Wall Bridge: Lie on your back, feet flat on the wall, knees bent. Lift your hips to the ceiling while focusing your glutes and core muscles, then hold for 30-60 seconds.

Women over 40 can benefit considerably from including transverse abdominis strengthening exercises in their training program, particularly via Wall Pilates sessions, because they improve core stability, posture, and general health.

Consistency and appropriate form are essential for attaining the best results and maintaining a strong, healthy physique as you age.

Spinal Articulation Exercises

spine articulation exercises are essential for preserving spine health and flexibility as we age, especially for women over 40. These exercises work the muscles that surround the spine, increasing mobility and stability along the whole vertebral column.

Here's a detailed guide on spinal articulation exercises, emphasizing their advantages and execution:

Benefits:

Improves spinal flexibility: Regular spinal articulation exercises serve to increase the range of motion in the spine, decreasing stiffness and facilitating better mobility.

Strengthens core muscles: These exercises work the core muscles, such as the abdominals and back, which are necessary for spine stability and appropriate posture.

Back pain relief: By strengthening the muscles that support the spine and fostering better alignment, spinal articulation exercises can help reduce back pain and prevent future suffering.

Improves posture: Strengthening and mobilizing the spine promotes improved posture, lowering the chance of developing postural disorders linked with age.

Execution:

Begin in a comfortable sitting or lying posture, with your spine in neutral alignment.
Start by breathing deeply, extending your chest, and filling your lungs with air.

As you exhale, start the movement with the lower spine, articulating each vertebra as you circle the spine into a C-curve.

Continue to exhale as you achieve the greatest flexion of your spine, utilizing your abdominal muscles to support the action.
Inhale to momentarily retain the position while using the core muscles.

Exhale as you reverse the action, stacking each vertebra to return to your starting position.

Repeat the exercise multiple times, focusing on smooth, controlled action throughout.

Wall Pilates Workouts for Women over 40:
Use a wall for further support and stability during Pilates workouts, which is especially useful for ladies over 40 who may require more spine support.

Integrate spinal articulation exercises into wall Pilates routines to optimize the advantages of both practices, with an emphasis on perfect alignment and controlled movement.

Begin with gentle variants of spinal articulation exercises against the wall, gradually increasing the intensity as your strength and flexibility increase.

Spinal articulation exercises, particularly when performed against a wall during Pilates workouts, can help women over 40 improve their spinal health and general well-being.

Chapter 4: Strength Training and Resistance Work

Strength training and resistance exercises are crucial components of a well-rounded fitness plan, especially for women over 40.

These workouts not only assist in growing muscular mass, but they also provide several health advantages, such as greater bone density, improved metabolism, improved joint function, and higher general functional strength.

Resistance training using weights or resistance bands is one of the most effective methods of building strength. This sort of training involves taxing the muscles with external resistance, which may be modified to meet individual fitness levels and goals.

Women over 40 may keep their muscles challenged and growing by gradually increasing resistance over time.

In addition to classic strength training exercises like squats, lunges, and deadlifts, women over 40 can benefit from using functional movements in their routines. These exercises simulate normal tasks and enhance balance, coordination, and stability, lowering the risk of falls and injury.

Wall Pilates routines provide a unique approach to strength training for ladies over 40. Pilates focuses on core strength, flexibility, and posture, making it especially effective for improving spinal health and relieving back pain, which can worsen with age.

Women may do a range of Pilates exercises with perfect alignment and form by utilizing the wall as a support, increasing their efficiency while lowering their risk of injury.

Some significant advantages of Wall Pilates workouts for women over 40 include:

Improved posture: Pilates movements target the muscles that support the spine, which helps to address postural imbalances and reduces the risk of back discomfort.

Increased flexibility: Because Wall Pilates workouts include dynamic stretching movements, they assist increase flexibility and range of motion, making daily tasks simpler and more pleasant.

Enhanced core strength: Strong core muscles are necessary for stability and balance, particularly as we age. Wall Pilates movements aim to develop the deep abdominal muscles, which serve to stabilize the spine and increase general core strength.

Wall Pilates movements are low-impact and soft on the joints, making them appropriate for women over 40 who may be experiencing joint discomfort or mobility concerns.

Strength training and resistance exercises, such as Wall Pilates sessions, are crucial for women over 40 who want to maintain muscle mass, bone density, and overall health.

Women who incorporate these exercises into their fitness program will benefit from increased strength, flexibility, and functional ability, resulting in a superior quality of life as they age.

Building Functional Strength

Functional strength is the foundation of physical fitness, particularly for women over 40 who want to retain their energy and independence as they age.

Unlike traditional strength training, which generally promotes heavy weight lifting, functional strength training focuses on exercises that imitate real-life motions and enhance daily functioning.

Building functional strength is important for women over 40 because it helps them feel strong in their bodies. It's about being able to carry groceries, hoist youngsters, and negotiate stairs with ease and confidence.

One effective approach to accomplish this is to perform focused workouts that activate numerous muscle groups while increasing mobility, stability, and flexibility.

Enter Wall Pilates routines, a versatile and accessible choice for women over 40 who want to improve their functional strength. These workouts use the support of a wall to give stability and aid, making them appropriate for people of various fitness levels and capabilities.

Wall Pilates focuses on core development. These exercises improve posture, spinal alignment, and general stability by targeting the deep abdominal muscles, obliques, and lower back. This not only relieves back discomfort but also lowers the likelihood of damage during regular activities.

Wall Pilates routines include balance and stability exercises, which are increasingly vital as we age. These exercises enhance balance and minimize the probability of falls by testing proprioception and coordination, which is especially important for women over 40.

Wall Pilates stresses utilitarian exercises that are directly applicable to daily work. Whether it's bending to pick up a laundry basket or reaching for something on a high shelf, these exercises train the body to move quickly and securely in everyday scenarios.

Wall Pilates practices rely on the mind-body connection that Pilates promotes. Women over 40 may increase their awareness of their bodies and have a better grasp of their physical skills by focusing on breath, concentration, and movement precision.

Building functional strength with Wall Pilates routines provides women over 40 with a comprehensive approach to training that promotes mobility, stability, and general health. These routines, which include core strengthening, balancing exercises, functional movements, and mindfulness methods, enable women to live actively and confidently at every stage of life. With consistency and effort, women over 40 may gain the multiple advantages of Wall Pilates, including increased strength, flexibility, and quality of life.

Wall Squats and Leg Press Variations

Wall squats and leg press variants are excellent workouts for increasing lower-body strength, stability, and muscular tone.

These exercises are especially beneficial for women over the age of 40 since they promote bone density, joint health, and functional fitness. To better comprehend the efficiency of each workout and its modifications, let's look at them individually.

Wall squats work the quadriceps, hamstrings, glutes, and core muscles. To execute a wall squat, stand with your back against a wall and your feet shoulder-width apart.

Slide down until your thighs are parallel to the ground, keeping your knees and ankles aligned. Hold this position for a few seconds before pushing back up to your starting position. Wall squat variations include placing a stability ball behind the back for additional support or carrying dumbbells for further resistance.

Leg press variants are another useful method for strengthening the lower body muscles. The classic leg press is performed on a machine by pushing a weighted platform away from your body with your legs.

This workout focuses largely on the quadriceps, hamstrings, and glutes. To provide diversity and difficulty, experiment with different foot locations on the leg press machine, such as narrow, broad, or high on the platform.

Each variant engages the muscles differently, resulting in a well-rounded lower-body exercise.

For women over 40, integrating wall squats and leg press variants into a regular workout regimen will help preserve bone density, which normally decreases with age.

Stronger muscles also promote joint health and lower the chance of injury, which is especially essential as we age and become more prone to conditions such as osteoarthritis.

These workouts increase balance and stability, which are critical for avoiding falls and retaining independence.

Incorporating Pilates techniques into wall squats can increase its efficacy for women over 40. Pilates emphasizes core strength, alignment, and mind-body connection, all of which promote general health and well-being.

Adding Pilates methods, like as activating the pelvic floor muscles and maintaining appropriate spinal alignment during wall squats, can increase their benefits while lowering the risk of strain or injury.

Wall squats and leg press variants are excellent workouts for women over 40 looking to increase their lower body strength, stability, and general health.

Women who incorporate these exercises into a well-rounded fitness regimen can maintain functional fitness, promote bone and joint health, and lead an active lifestyle for many years.

Upper Body Resistance Training using the Wall

Upper body resistance training against a wall is an excellent and simple approach to building and toning muscles, especially for women over 40. Wall Pilates workouts have various advantages, including improved posture, muscle strength, stability, and total functional fitness.

One of the most significant benefits of using the wall for resistance training is that it provides a sturdy surface to work against, allowing for controlled motions and appropriate alignment. This is especially helpful for women over 40, who may be more prone to injury or have unique mobility issues.

Wall exercises can work for numerous muscular groups in the upper body, including the chest, back, shoulders, arms, and core. Popular workouts include wall push-ups, wall angels, wall slides, wall sits with arm reaches, and wall planks. These exercises are adaptable to all fitness levels and skills, making them suitable for both beginners and expert practitioners.

Regular upper body strength training on the wall can assist women over 40 prevent age-related muscle loss, often known as sarcopenia. Individuals who challenge their muscles against resistance can maintain or develop muscular mass and strength, resulting in better overall health and functionality.

Wall Pilates routines provide a low-impact option for anyone with joint problems or restricted mobility. The wall offers support and stability, allowing people to exercise with appropriate form and technique while putting less strain on their joints.

Wall resistance training, when combined with a full exercise plan, can improve upper-body flexibility and range of motion. Stretching and lengthening exercises, such as wall angels and wall slides, serve to enhance joint mobility and reduce stiffness, which is especially useful as we age.

Wall Pilates routines may be readily included in a home training regimen, requiring little equipment and space. All that is required is a clear wall surface and maybe a yoga mat for enhanced comfort.

This accessibility enables women over 40 to prioritize their fitness and include regular strength training in their hectic lives. Upper body resistance training against the wall, particularly through Pilates routines, has various benefits for women over 40.

Wall exercises offer a comprehensive solution for maintaining optimal upper body health and functionality, ranging from muscular strength and posture to stability and flexibility.

Incorporating Resistance Bands for Added Challenge

Incorporating resistance bands into wall Pilates routines can improve their efficacy and difficulty, particularly for women over 40. These bands offer varied resistance, allowing for specific muscle engagement and general strength development. Here's a detailed tutorial on using resistance bands in wall Pilates workouts:

Warm-Up: Start with a quick warm-up to get your body ready for a workout. To promote blood flow and flexibility, do dynamic motions like arm circles, leg swings, and torso twists.

Choose the Right Bands: Select resistance bands with the proper strength for your fitness level. Beginners can start with lesser bands and move to stronger ones as their strength increases.

Secure Anchoring: Attach the resistance band firmly to a wall-mounted fixture or a strong door frame. Ensure that the band is at the proper height for the workouts you'll be doing.

Upper Body Exercises: Use tension bands for bicep curls, shoulder presses, and chest flies. The bands maintain consistent tension throughout the activity, increasing muscle activation and strength.

Lower Body Exercises: Use resistance bands to perform squats, lunges, and leg lifts. These motions strengthen the legs and glutes while also improving balance and stability.

Strengthen your core muscles with workouts including standing side bends, wood chops, and torso twists using resistance bands.

These actions serve to stabilize the spine and enhance posture.

Mindful Movement: Maintain good form and alignment during each exercise to avoid injury and optimize efficacy. Pay close attention to the muscles being targeted and keep control of the resistance band at all times.

Progressive Overload: As your strength and endurance develop, gradually increase the resistance or repetitions. This gradual overburden is necessary for ongoing development and adaptability.

Cool Down and Stretch: Finish your wall Pilates exercise with a cooldown and stretching practice to enhance recovery and flexibility. Stretch the muscles that were worked during the training for 15-30 seconds apiece.

Incorporating resistance bands into wall Pilates sessions provides women over 40 with a diverse and difficult technique to improve strength, stability, and general fitness. With good technique and consistency, you may significantly enhance muscular tone, endurance, and functional mobility.

Chapter 5: Balance and Stability Training

As women age, keeping balance and stability becomes more crucial for their general health and well-being. Balance and stability training are essential components of any comprehensive fitness plan, particularly for women over 40.

These exercises not only serve to prevent falls and injuries, but also improve posture, mobility, and confidence in everyday tasks. Among the different approaches available, Wall Pilates Workouts stand out as especially effective for women in this demographic, as they provide tailored exercises to improve balance and stability while using the support of a wall.

Let's look at the importance of balance and stability training for women over 40, and how Wall Pilates Workouts may help them achieve these goals.

Why Does Balance and Stability Training Matter?

A loss in balance and stability can occur as people age due to a variety of circumstances. These include changes in muscular strength, joint flexibility, eyesight, and proprioception (the body's capacity to perceive its location in space). Without effective care, impaired balance and stability can result in falls, fractures, and loss of independence.

Balance and stability training tackles these difficulties by focusing on specific muscle groups that help maintain equilibrium and control. Individuals who incorporate workouts that stress balance and coordination might enhance their ability to react to unexpected movements, manage uneven terrain, and maintain equilibrium in a variety of settings.

Balance and stability exercise is especially beneficial to women over the age of 40. Menopause-related hormonal changes can reduce bone density and muscle mass, increasing the risk of osteoporosis and frailty.

Lifestyle choices such as less physical exercise and extended sitting can worsen muscular weakness and postural abnormalities.

Women over 40 who incorporate balance and stability exercises into their workout program can reduce these risks while also promoting long-term health and vitality.

Improved balance not only lowers the risk of falls and accidents but also improves overall quality of life by allowing people to participate in activities they like with confidence and ease.

The Role of Wall Pilates Workouts

Wall Pilates Workouts provide a unique approach to balance and stability training by combining Pilates concepts with the extra stability of a wall.

Pilates focuses on core strength, flexibility, and body awareness, giving it an excellent basis for balance training. By using the wall as a support, people may do exercises with better control and accuracy, making them accessible to people of all fitness levels.

These workouts generally consist of a sequence of standing, sitting, and reclining movements meant to test balance while encouraging appropriate alignment and posture. Individuals who use the wall for support may focus on engaging the core, activating stabilizing muscles, and developing proprioception without worry of falling.

Wall Pilates Workouts are extremely versatile, allowing people to go at their speed and alter exercises to meet their specific needs. Whether you're doing leg lifts, squats, or arm reaches, the wall provides a firm surface to help you balance while promoting good form.

Balance and stability training are critical components of a well-rounded fitness program, especially for women over 40. Individuals who incorporate workouts that stress balance and control might improve their ability to handle daily tasks with confidence and comfort.

Wall Pilates Workouts provide a safe and effective technique to develop balance and stability while also increasing general strength and flexibility. Women may receive the advantages of Pilates-based exercises while maintaining safety and efficacy by using a wall as support. With regularity and attention, balance and stability training may help women live active, independent lives far into their elderly years.

Finding Your Center

Finding your center is essential on the path to wellness and fitness, especially for women over 40 looking for long-term solutions to stay healthy and strong. Wall Pilates routines provide a holistic approach that emphasizes both physical strength and mental balance, making them an excellent choice for women in this group.

Wall Pilates is based on classic Pilates concepts but uses a wall for support and resistance. This novel technique provides stability, allowing users to concentrate on perfect alignment and form while doing a variety of activities.

This is especially advantageous to women over 40 since it reduces the chance of injury and promotes joint health. One of the most important parts of establishing your center with Wall Pilates is the emphasis on core strength.

As we become older, having a strong core becomes more crucial for general stability and posture. Wall Pilates focuses on the deep abdominal muscles, pelvic floor, and back muscles, promoting core strength and stability, which is necessary for everyday tasks and preventing back problems.

Wall Pilates practices also integrate mindfulness and breath awareness. This comprehensive approach improves not just physical strength but also mental clarity and calm. For women over 40 who are coping with the demands of the job, family, and other commitments, this part of Wall Pilates may be quite beneficial in promoting a feeling of balance and well-being.

Wall Pilates sessions are highly adaptable to varied fitness levels and personal preferences. Whether you're a novice or have been doing Pilates for years, some routines and variations will challenge and engage you at your speed.

Finding your core with Wall Pilates routines provides several benefits to ladies over 40. This complete approach to training serves the special demands of this group by strengthening core strength and posture while also fostering mental clarity and relaxation.

 By including Wall Pilates into your regimen, you may develop a strong, balanced body and mind that will help you live your life to the fullest.

Single-Leg Stances with Wall Support

Single-leg stances with wall support are an excellent complement to Pilates routines, especially for women over 40 aiming to increase their balance, stability, and general strength. This exercise works the core, and lower body muscles, and improves proprioception.

To begin the single-leg stance with wall support, stand with your side facing a wall. Place one hand lightly on the wall for support. Lift one leg off the ground, bending the knee while keeping the supporting leg slightly bent.

To keep your body stable, use your core muscles. Hold this stance for 15-30 seconds and then swap legs. To make this workout more challenging, close your eyes or hold the posture for a longer period. As you advance, consider lowering the amount of support from the wall until you can complete the exercise without help.

The advantages of single-leg postures with wall support include:

Improved Balance: Standing on one leg while maintaining stability against the wall tests your balance and proprioception, both of which are essential for avoiding falls and accidents, especially as you become older.

Lower Body Strengthening: This workout focuses on leg muscles such as the quadriceps, hamstrings, and calves, as well as stabilizing muscles around the ankles and hips, to assist enhance total lower body strength.

Enhanced Core Stability: Using the core muscles to maintain balance in a single-leg stance improves the abdominals, obliques, and lower back muscles, resulting in improved posture and spinal alignment.

Functional Fitness: Practicing single-leg stances with wall support simulates real-life actions like walking, climbing stairs, and reaching for things while standing on one leg, making it a functional workout that leads to better everyday activities.

Injury Prevention: By strengthening muscles and improving balance, this exercise can help minimize the risk of common injuries like ankle sprains and knee strains, especially in women over 40, who are more prone to age-related muscle and joint problems.

Incorporating single-leg stances with wall support into a daily Pilates program may result in significant improvements in balance, stability, and general fitness, making it a crucial exercise for women over 40 looking to stay active and healthy.

Proprioceptive Challenges for Balance

Proprioceptive problems for balance are severe, particularly for women over 40 who participate in Wall Pilates routines. Proprioception is the body's capacity to perceive its position, movement, and spatial orientation. As we age, this capacity deteriorates, making balancing exercises critical for maintaining equilibrium and avoiding falls.

Wall Pilates workouts present unique proprioceptive difficulties because they use the support and resistance offered by a wall. These workouts benefit women over 40 by improving balance, coordination, and muscular strength while lowering the chance of injury.

One major proprioceptive challenge in Wall Pilates is keeping good alignment and stability against the wall. This necessitates increased awareness of body alignment and muscle engagement.

Individuals must rely on proprioceptive cues to guarantee proper form and balance when performing exercises against the wall, such as squats, lunges, or leg lifts. Another problem is altering weight distribution while remaining stable. During varied activities, participants must continually change their center of gravity, depending on proprioceptive signals to maintain balance.

Wall Pilates workouts frequently include dynamic movements, such as reaching or twisting actions, which test proprioception. To be effective, these motions must be executed with exact synchronization and control while remaining stable against the wall.

Wall Pilates incorporates props such as stability balls or resistance bands, which adds another degree of proprioceptive challenge. Balancing on an unstable surface or resisting external pressures increases proprioceptive input, which improves general balance and stability.

Wall Pilates sessions with proprioceptive difficulties offer several benefits to women over 40. Improved balance not only lowers the chance of falls and injuries, but also improves everyday functional activities like walking or climbing stairs.

 improved proprioception can lead to better posture and body awareness, which promotes general physical health.
Proprioceptive difficulties are essential to Wall Pilates routines, particularly for women over 40. Individuals can increase proprioception, minimize the chance of falls, and improve overall physical performance

and well-being by implementing workouts that focus on balance, coordination, and muscle control against the support of a wall.

Core Stability Exercises with Wall Assistance

Wall Pilates routines provide excellent support and stability for ladies over 40 who want to build their core muscles efficiently.

These workouts are particularly intended to focus on the core while using the wall as support, creating a safe and regulated setting for people of all fitness levels. Here are some complete core stability exercises with a wall aid designed for ladies over 40:

Wall Plank: Face the wall and place your hands shoulder-width apart against it. Walk your feet back until your body forms a straight line from head to heels, then engage your core muscles. Hold this posture for 30-60 seconds, keeping your abs strong and your back flat against the wall.

Wall Sit: Stand with your back against the wall and lower yourself into a seated position, as if in an imaginary chair. Keep your knees bent at a 90-degree angle and your back placed firmly against the wall. Maintain this position for 30-60 seconds, feeling the heat in your quadriceps and core muscles.

Wall Bridge: Lie on your back, feet flat on the wall, knees bent at a 90-degree angle. Press your lower back into the floor while lifting your hips to the ceiling, forming a straight line from your shoulders to your knees. Hold this position for 15 to 30 seconds, squeezing your glutes and working your core.

Wall Knee Tucks: Begin in a high plank posture, facing away from the wall, with your hands shoulder-width apart on the floor. Put your feet against the wall, hip-width apart. Draw your knees towards your chest and move your feet up the wall while engaging your core. Extend your legs back to the beginning position and repeat 10-15 times, concentrating on controlled motions.

Wall Side Plank: Lie on your side, forearm on the floor, and feet against the wall, stacking them on top of each other. Lift your hips off the floor to form a straight line from head to heels. Hold this position for 20-30 seconds, concentrating on core stability and preventing hip rotation.

Incorporating these core stability exercises with wall aid into your Pilates regimen will help women over 40 increase their strength, stability, and general fitness. Remember to keep appropriate form and alignment during each exercise to optimize efficacy and avoid injury.

Chapter 6: Enhancing Flexibility and Mobility

Improving flexibility and mobility is critical for women over 40 to maintain good health and well-being. Wall Pilates workouts provide an efficient and easy approach to reaching these objectives.

Pilates emphasizes core strength, flexibility, and body awareness, making it an excellent training program for ladies looking to improve their flexibility and mobility. Women over 40 can enhance the advantages of Pilates by including the wall in their workouts.

One of the primary benefits of Wall Pilates workouts is the additional support and stability offered by the wall. This is especially advantageous for ladies over the age of 40 who may struggle with balance or are concerned about their safety while exercising. The wall acts as a guide, allowing for perfect alignment while lowering the chance of harm.

Wall Pilates movements may also address parts of the body that lose flexibility and mobility as we age, such as the spine, hips, and shoulders.

Women over 40 can enhance their range of motion and joint mobility in these areas by using the wall for support and resistance, thus increasing total flexibility and lowering stiffness.

Wall Pilates routines provide a diverse approach to training, with exercises that can be readily adapted to suit various fitness levels and individual demands.

Women over 40 may customize their exercises to meet their unique objectives and interests, whether they like mild stretches or more strenuous activities.

Consistency is essential for improving flexibility and mobility, and Wall Pilates routines are a handy way to include regular exercise into a busy lifestyle. Women over 40 may easily include Wall Pilates into their daily regimen because it requires minimum equipment and allows them to conduct various exercises from the comfort of their own homes.

Wall Pilates routines provide a thorough and effective technique for women over 40 to improve flexibility and mobility. Women can enhance their range of motion, joint mobility, and general physical well-being by using the wall as support and integrating focused exercises.

With consistent practice, Wall Pilates may help women over 40 feel stronger, more nimble, and more prepared to live an active and rewarding life.

Lengthening and Loosening

Lengthening and relaxing are key elements in Wall Pilates routines, especially for ladies over 40. These exercises are designed particularly for adult bodies, to increase flexibility, posture, and strength. Let's go into these two critical aspects:

Lengthening: wall Pilates focuses on lengthening muscles to improve alignment and range of motion. As women age, their muscles shorten and contract, resulting in stiffness and diminished mobility.

Gentle stretches and motions are used to lengthen key muscular groups such as the hamstrings, quadriceps, back, and shoulders. Participants can reduce stress, avoid accidents, and increase general flexibility by lengthening these muscles.

Loosening is the process of relieving tension and stiffness in the body, especially in areas prone to tightness as a result of sedentary lifestyles or repetitive activities. Wall Pilates uses a variety of methods, including myofascial release and dynamic stretching, to loosen tight muscles and fascia.

Foam rolling against the wall, for example, aids in the breakdown of adhesions and knots, whilst dynamic stretches such as leg swings and arm circles enhance circulation and relax tight joints.

These ideas are especially useful for women over the age of 40, who experience physiological changes as they age.

Lengthening and loosening exercises can help counteract the consequences of muscle loss, joint stiffness, and reduced flexibility that are prevalent with age.

Women who incorporate these aspects into their workouts can retain mobility, avoid injury, and improve general well-being.

Wall Pilates routines use a wall to help participants maintain stability and alignment while executing movements. This creates a safe and productive setting for women over 40 to practice strength and flexibility training.

The use of props like resistance bands and stability balls offers variation and difficulty to exercises, increasing their efficacy.

Wall Pilates routines for women over 40 include lengthening and relaxing exercises. Participants who prioritize these components might enjoy more flexibility, less muscular strain, and better overall function.

As women age, incorporating these concepts into a regular exercise regimen might help them improve their posture, mobility, and quality of life.

Upper Body Stretching Against the Wall

As women become older, maintaining flexibility and mobility in the upper body becomes more crucial for their general health and well-being. Incorporating wall

Pilates routines into your program will help you gain flexibility and decrease stress. In this complete tutorial, we'll look at upper body stretching exercises against a wall intended exclusively for ladies over 40.

Importance of Upper Body Stretching

Before beginning the exercises, it's critical to understand why upper body stretching is so important, particularly for women over 40. Muscles tend to tighten as we age, resulting in less flexibility and an increased risk of injury.

Regular stretching helps to combat this by increasing range of motion, decreasing muscular stiffness, and maintaining good posture.

Benefits of Wall Pilates Workout

Wall Pilates routines provide various benefits, especially for women over 40. These exercises stretch and develop the upper body safely and effectively by utilizing the wall as support and resistance.

Additionally, wall Pilates can assist increase balance, stability, and core strength, all of which are necessary for preserving independence and avoiding falls as we age.

Upper Body Stretching Exercises.

Wall Chest Stretch: Stand facing a wall, feet hip-width apart. Place your palms flat on the wall, shoulder height and a little wider than shoulder width apart. Lean forward and feel a nice stretch over your chest and shoulders.

Release after holding for a period of 20-30 seconds

Wall Shoulder Stretch: Stand sideways next to a wall, your left shoulder facing it. Reach your left arm across your body, palm flat against the wall at shoulder level. Gently twist your body away from the wall, feeling a stretch in your shoulder and upper back. Hold for 20-30 seconds and then swap sides.

Wall Upper Back Stretch: Stand facing away from the wall and extend your arms straight out in front of you, palms flat against the wall, shoulder height. Slowly move your feet backward until your arms are completely extended and your body is in a straight line from head to heels.

Push your chest to the floor, experiencing a stretch in your upper back and shoulders. Hold for 20 to 30 seconds.

Wall Triceps Stretch: Stand facing the wall, lift your right arm overhead, bend your elbow, and extend your hand to the center of your back. Using your left hand, gently press your right elbow against the wall until you feel a triceps stretch. Hold for 20-30 seconds and then swap sides.

Wall Neck Stretch: Stand with your right side facing the wall and lay your right hand against the wall at shoulder level.

Tilt your head to the left, putting your left ear close to your left shoulder, until you feel a stretch on the right side of your neck. Hold for 20-30 seconds and then swap sides.

Tips for Safe and Effective Stretching.
Before you begin, warm up your muscles with some mild aerobic or dynamic stretches.

Move slowly and carefully into each stretch, avoiding any abrupt or jerky movements.

The capabilities of your body should not be pushed beyond its limit, relax into the stretch after Breathing deeply

Hold each stretch for 20-30 seconds, progressively increasing the duration with time.

Listen to your body and adjust the workouts to meet any restrictions or injuries.
Incorporating these upper body stretching exercises against the wall into your daily routine will help you improve your flexibility, decrease stress, and feel better overall.

To get the most advantages, execute them regularly and with appropriate form. Stay consistent and you'll quickly see the benefits of wall Pilates routines for women over 40.

Lower Body Release Techniques

Lower body release methods are vital for women over 40 who participate in wall Pilates exercises to improve flexibility, mobility, and general health.

These techniques aim to relieve tension, stiffness, and discomfort in the lower body, namely the hips, thighs, and calves.

Foam rolling is an efficient lower-body release method. Using a foam roller, ladies may target particular areas of tension by rolling it back and forth beneath their hips, thighs, and calves.

This self-myofascial release technique helps to break up muscular adhesions and knots, resulting in improved blood flow and range of motion.

Another useful approach is static stretching. Women can relieve stiffness and increase lower-body flexibility by performing mild stretches for their hamstrings, quadriceps, hip flexors, and calf muscles. Incorporating static stretches into a wall Pilates practice can help minimize injury and increase training efficacy.

Additionally, including mobility exercises within the regimen helps improve lower body release. Leg swings, hip circles, and ankle circles are all dynamic motions that serve to release tight muscles and joints, hence increasing general mobility and function.

Trigger point treatment can be utilized to relieve stress in specific parts of the lower body. Women can easily relieve muscle tension and soreness by applying focused pressure to trigger points with a lacrosse ball or massage ball against a wall.

It's critical to incorporate these lower body release methods into a full wall Pilates training regimen. Women over 40 may maximize their exercises by combining strength, flexibility, and release methods to obtain better muscular tone, posture, and general fitness.

Lower body release methods are vital for ladies over 40 who engage in wall Pilates sessions. These techniques serve to relieve stiffness, tension, and discomfort in the lower body, enhancing flexibility, mobility, and general well-being.

 Women who incorporate foam rolling, static stretching, mobility exercises, and trigger point treatment into their routine can improve the efficacy of their workouts and obtain greater outcomes in terms of strength, flexibility, and general fitness.

Spinal Mobility Drills

Spinal mobility drills are essential for women over 40 who participate in Wall Pilates Workouts to promote flexibility, posture improvement, and injury avoidance. These workouts, designed exclusively for spinal health, strengthen the backbone's range of motion, assuring peak functionality. Here's an in-depth look at spinal mobility drills:

1. Cat-Cow Stretch: Begin on all fours, hands beneath shoulders, knees aligned under hips. Inhale deeply, arching your back and elevating your head and tailbone upwards to simulate a cow's stance.

Exhale gently, rounding the spine and tucking the chin towards the chest like a stretched cat. Iterating these motions numerous times releases and mobilizes the whole spine, reducing tension and increasing flexibility.

2. *Seated Spinal Twist:* Sit with legs outstretched and maintain an erect posture. Bend one knee and place the foot on the outside of the opposing thigh. Inhale deeply, lengthening the spine, then exhale to begin a slight twist towards the bent knee.

Place the opposite hand on the knee to provide leverage, while the other hand supports the twist by resting behind the back. Holding this position for a few breaths on each side promotes spine flexibility and relieves accumulated stress.

3. *Child's Pose:* Begin in a tabletop posture, then gently drop the hips to the heels while extending the arms forward and resting the forehead on the ground. This restorative position stretches the spine, hips, and thighs, promoting relaxation and increasing spinal flexibility.

4. *Standing Side Bend:* Stand tall, feet hip-width apart, arms extended overhead, and hands clasped. Inhale deeply to lengthen the spine, then exhale and slowly lean to one side while feeling a stretch down the opposing side of the body.

Return to the middle and do the motion on the other side. This lateral stretch improves spine mobility and alleviates stiffness.

5. *Bridge Pose:* Begin lying on your back with knees bent and feet hip-width apart. Press hard onto your feet, elevating your hips to the ceiling and working your glutes and core.

Hold the pose for a few breaths, enjoying the stretch across the chest and strengthening your back muscles. Bridge Pose, after lowering back down, strengthens the spine's stability and increases mobility.

6. *Thread the Needle:* Start on all fours, then snake one arm beneath the opposing arm, dropping the shoulder and temple to the ground.

Hold this pose for a few breaths to feel a deep stretch in the upper back and shoulders. Next, repeat the technique on the opposite side. Thread the Needle improves spine flexibility and relieves strain from sedentary lifestyles.

Incorporating these spinal mobility activities into Wall Pilates Workouts for Women Over 40 helps to improve flexibility, refine movement quality, and strengthen spinal health.

Regular practice of these exercises improves posture and reduces stiffness, promoting a greater appreciation for daily tasks. For best results, tailor workouts to your requirements and skills, and pay close attention to your body's indications.

Chapter 7: Progressing Your Practice

As women age past 40, the desire for health and vitality becomes increasingly important. Among the variety of training alternatives, Wall Pilates stands out as a beacon of strength, flexibility, and rejuvenation. It provides a transforming path to overall well-being, allowing women to move forward with confidence.

Strength and Stability: Wall Pilates is essential for developing core strength and stability. As women age, preserving muscle mass becomes increasingly important for general health.

Pilates routines target deep abdominal muscles by using the wall's resistance to improve stability and posture. This enhanced power boosts women's confidence, allowing them to face daily problems with ease.

Flexibility and Mobility: Embracing the Wall Pilates promotes flexibility and mobility, both of which are crucial for elegant aging.

Participants progressively relieve tension and tightness via gentle stretches and regulated movements, allowing them to move more freely. Improved flexibility not only improves physical performance but also fosters mental relaxation, resulting in a sense of peace and clarity.

Mind-Body Connection: Center to Wall Pilates focuses on developing the mind-body connection. By stressing mindful movement and breath awareness, practitioners get a better knowledge of their bodies.

This increased awareness allows women to move with intention and accuracy, lowering their risk of injury and optimizing the advantages of each activity. The synergy of mind and body promotes empowerment, allowing women to manage life's transitions with grace and fortitude.

Community and Support: Participating in Wall Pilates fosters a sense of community and support among like-minded people.

Shared experiences and mutual encouragement motivate women to continue their fitness journey, celebrating milestones and conquering hurdles together. This sense of belonging boosts confidence by ensuring that one is not alone in their pursuit of health and vitality.

Embracing Change: When women join Wall Pilates, they begin a journey of self-discovery and change. By accepting change and venturing beyond their comfort zones, people realize latent potential and welcome new opportunities. Each Pilates class helps women develop a sense of empowerment and resilience, giving them the courage to meet life's obstacles head-on.

Wall Pilates can help women over 40 go forward with confidence. Through strength, flexibility, awareness, and community, it enables women to accept their path with grace and energy, embracing the spirit of empowered aging.

Advanced Wall Pilates Techniques

Wall Pilates is a versatile and effective exercise that uses the assistance of a wall to improve stability, alignment, and strength.

Advanced Wall Pilates methods are specifically designed for women over 40, providing a complete approach to enhancing general fitness, mobility, and body awareness. Let's look at the foundational ideas and main exercises of this inspiring training plan.

1. Core Stability and Alignment:

Wall Pilates focuses on core stability and alignment. Women over 40 who use the deep muscles of the belly, back, and pelvis can improve their posture, relieve back pain, and improve general spinal health.

Pelvic tilts, spinal articulation, and imprinting are all techniques that help to achieve ideal alignment and support.

2. Functional Movement Patterns:

As women become older, keeping functional mobility becomes more crucial for everyday tasks and injury avoidance. Advanced Wall Pilates techniques include functional movement patterns in workouts including squats, lunges, and rotations. These motions are designed to simulate real-life tasks while also improving strength, balance, and coordination.

3. Joint mobility and flexibility:

Aging can cause stiffness and reduced joint mobility, therefore flexibility exercise is vital for women over 40. Wall Pilates uses dynamic stretches and range-of-motion movements to increase joint mobility and flexibility. Techniques such as shoulder circles, leg swings, and spinal twists improve mobility while lowering the chance of injury.

4. Balance and proprioception:

Maintaining balance and proprioception is essential for fall prevention and general stability, particularly as women age. Advanced Wall Pilates techniques incorporate balancing problems with the help of the wall. Exercises like single-leg stands, heel lifts, and stability ball presses improve balance, proprioception, and spatial awareness.

5. Strength and endurance:

Building strength and endurance are essential components of any successful fitness program, especially for women over 40. Advanced Wall Pilates routines include bodyweight resistance, resistance bands, and tiny props to target particular muscle regions. Exercises like wall push-ups, leg lifts, and side planks help to improve the upper, lower, and core muscles.

6. Mind-Body Connections:

Wall Pilates emphasizes mindfulness and body awareness, which promotes mental relaxation and stress alleviation. Advanced approaches include breathing exercises, visualization, and mindful movement to improve the mind-body connection. Practicing breath and movement awareness helps you feel peaceful and present during your exercises.

7. Progress and Variation:

Advanced Wall Pilates techniques focus on development and variation to keep the body challenged and prevent plateaus. Women over 40 can continue to enhance their strength, flexibility, and general fitness levels by gradually increasing the intensity, introducing new exercises, and using equipment.

8. Injury Prevention and Rehab:

For women over the age of 40, injury prevention and recovery are top priorities. Advanced Wall Pilates techniques provide low-impact workouts that develop joint stability and muscle balance while reducing stress on the body. In addition, Wall Pilates may be utilized as a rehabilitation technique to help people recover from injuries or surgery.

Advanced Wall Pilates methods give women over 40 a thorough and successful training plan that targets their specific fitness goals. Wall Pilates takes a comprehensive approach to enhancing total health and well-being, emphasizing core stability, functional movement, flexibility, balance, strength, mindfulness, progression, and injury prevention. Whether practiced at home or in a studio, adding these advanced methods into a daily training regimen may result in considerable gains in strength, mobility, and vitality.

Customizing Workouts for Individual Needs

Customizing exercises to individual needs is critical for attaining the best outcomes, particularly for women over 40 who participate in activities such as Wall Pilates. Tailoring workouts to personal needs improves safety, efficacy, and enjoyment. Here is a complete guide on tailoring Wall Pilates programs for ladies over 40:

Start by examining the person's fitness level, health issues, and aspirations. This examination assists in determining the right intensity, duration, and exercise kinds to include.

Focus on Core Strength: As women age, core strength becomes increasingly important for stability, posture, and overall health. Planks, pelvic tilts, and leg lifts are examples of core-targeting workouts that can help with stability and spine health.

Balance and Coordination: Aging can impair balance and coordination, raising the risk of falling. Balance-enhancing activities such as single-leg stands, heel-to-toe walks, and stability ball motions can help enhance proprioception and lower the chance of injury.

Flexibility and mobility tend to decline with age, resulting in stiffness and a limited range of motion. Incorporate stretching exercises into your regimen to increase flexibility, relieve stress, and improve joint mobility. Concentrate on regions prone to tension, such as the hips, hamstrings, and shoulders.

Low-impact workouts and joint-friendly motions are recommended to accommodate any existing joint difficulties or disorders, such as arthritis. Choose exercises that are easy on the joints while yet delivering a good workout, such as sitting variants, mild stretches, and controlled motions.

Progressive Overload: Gradually increase the intensity, length, or resistance of your exercises over time to push your body and encourage continual development. This progressive overload technique eliminates plateaus and assures consistent fitness increases.

Mind-Body Connection: Incorporate mindfulness and relaxation techniques into your exercises to reduce stress, promote mental health, and strengthen the mind-body connection. Deep breathing, visualization, and meditation techniques can be used in conjunction with physical activity to promote overall health and vitality.

Personalization: Tailor the exercises to the individual's tastes, interests, and limits. Encourage experimenting with new exercises, equipment, and forms to keep the workouts interesting and fun.

Individuals who customize Wall Pilates programs to match the special demands of women over 40 can find increased fitness, well-being, and energy in their everyday lives.

Maintaining Consistency and Long-Term Progress

Consistency is the foundation of development, particularly in Wall Pilates programs designed for women over 40.

These routines, which aim to enhance strength, flexibility, and general well-being, need dedication and perseverance for long-term results. Let's look at how consistency adds to long-term improvement in Wall Pilates programs for this group.

Understanding the importance of consistency:

Consistency is the foundation of every fitness regimen, and Wall Pilates exercises are no exception. Women over 40 who engage in these exercises regularly can receive a variety of advantages, including greater core strength, better posture, increased flexibility, and a lower chance of injury. Consistency not only increases the effectiveness of each session but also promotes habit development, making it simpler to stick to the training routine over time.

Setting realistic goals:o

To retain consistency, create reasonable and attainable goals. For women over 40, these aims may include improving mobility, relieving back discomfort, or increasing general fitness.

Individuals may stay motivated and measure their progress by setting specific goals, which fosters a sense of success and supports continuous consistency in their Wall Pilates practice.

Create a Structured Routine:

Consistency thrives in structured environments. Creating a regular training routine allows you to smoothly integrate Wall Pilates sessions into your everyday life. An organized program, whether it involves setting out certain days and times for exercise or introducing shorter, more frequent exercises into the week, instills discipline and ensures that consistency becomes a habit rather than a random effort.

Listen to Your Body:

While consistency is key, it's also important to listen to your body and alter your routines accordingly, especially as you get older. Women over 40 may suffer changes in strength, flexibility, and energy levels, necessitating adjustments to their Wall Pilates programs.

Honoring these bodily cues not only minimizes injury but also promotes a long-term attitude to training by encouraging consistency and improvement.

Embracing variety

Maintaining consistency does not imply boredom. Adding diversity to Wall Pilates sessions keeps them interesting and avoids boredom or plateaus.

Experimenting with different exercises, equipment, or workout forms not only challenges the body in new ways but also stimulates the mind, reviving motivation and passion for regular practice.

Seeking professional guidance:

For women over 40 starting Wall Pilates routines, receiving expert advice from trained instructors or physical therapists is crucial.

These specialists may customize workouts to meet individual needs, address any worries or limits, and offer continuing support and encouragement. Individuals may approach their Pilates practice with confidence thanks to their instruction, which promotes consistency and long-term growth.

Prioritizing Recovery and Rest.

Consistency does not imply pushing the body to its limits without rest. Prioritizing recuperation and relaxation is critical to avoiding burnout and maintaining long-term growth.

Including rest days in the weekly schedule, practicing easy stretching or relaxation methods, and getting enough sleep all help to good recuperation, allowing women over 40 to approach their Wall Pilates sessions with fresh zest and regularity.

Developing a Positive Mindset:

Consistency thrives in a good mentality. Cultivating self-compassion, patience, and resilience creates a helpful inner dialogue that pulls people onward, even in the face of failures or problems. Women over 40 may maintain enthusiasm and dedication to their Wall Pilates practice in the long run by viewing challenges as opportunities for growth and enjoying minor victories.

Maintaining consistency in Wall Pilates routines for women over 40 is critical for gaining long-term improvement and receiving the numerous advantages these exercises provide.

Individuals can establish long-term habits that promote health, vitality, and well-being by setting realistic goals, developing a structured routine, listening to their bodies, embracing variety, seeking professional advice, prioritizing recovery, and cultivating a positive mindset.

CONCLUSION

Wall Pilates routines provide several advantages targeted exclusively for women over 40, addressing their unique physiological demands and lifestyle problems.

A thorough examination of the ideas and exercises related to wall Pilates reveals that this kind of exercise is a safe, effective, and accessible method for improving general health and well-being.

First and foremost, wall Pilates encourages better posture and core strength, which are especially important for women over 40, who may face age-related changes in musculature and bone alignment.

Using the wall as support allows participants to better activate their abdominal muscles and spinal stabilizers, resulting in improved spinal alignment and a lower chance of injury. This is especially useful for treating common problems like lower back discomfort and postural abnormalities, which grow increasingly common with age.

Wall Pilates is a low-impact kind of exercise that is mild on the joints, making it appropriate for people with arthritis or other joint-related illnesses common in women over 40.

The regulated motions and emphasis on breathwork also assist in enhancing flexibility and mobility, counteracting the stiffness and limited range of motion that are commonly linked with aging.

The adaptability of wall Pilates allows for countless changes and adjustments to suit people of all fitness levels and abilities. Participants may modify their workouts to meet their unique requirements and goals by completing standing exercises, sitting motions, or using props like resistance bands and stability balls. This versatility makes wall Pilates an accessible and sustainable kind of exercise that can be readily incorporated into daily activities.

In addition to its physical advantages, wall Pilates supports mental health by encouraging awareness, relaxation, and stress reduction.

The emphasis on breath awareness and mindful movement enables practitioners to be in the now, resulting in a sensation of serenity and mental clarity.

For women over 40 who are juggling several obligations and feeling high levels of stress, including wall Pilates into their routine can give a much-needed outlet for self-care and refreshment.

Wall Pilates routines provide a comprehensive approach to fitness and well-being for women over the age of 40, addressing both physical and emotional health.

Wall Pilates, which incorporates concepts of alignment, core strength, flexibility, and mindfulness, enables people to maintain vigor, resilience, and a strong sense of vitality while aging.

THANK YOU PAGE

Thank you for selecting this book. Your support is really appreciated. Similarly, I am grateful for the purchase of this book.

Your input is valuable; please share your ideas in a review. It serves as a reference for future improvements. Enjoy reading and utilizing it!

*Workout planner
to help track
progress and
improvements
over time*

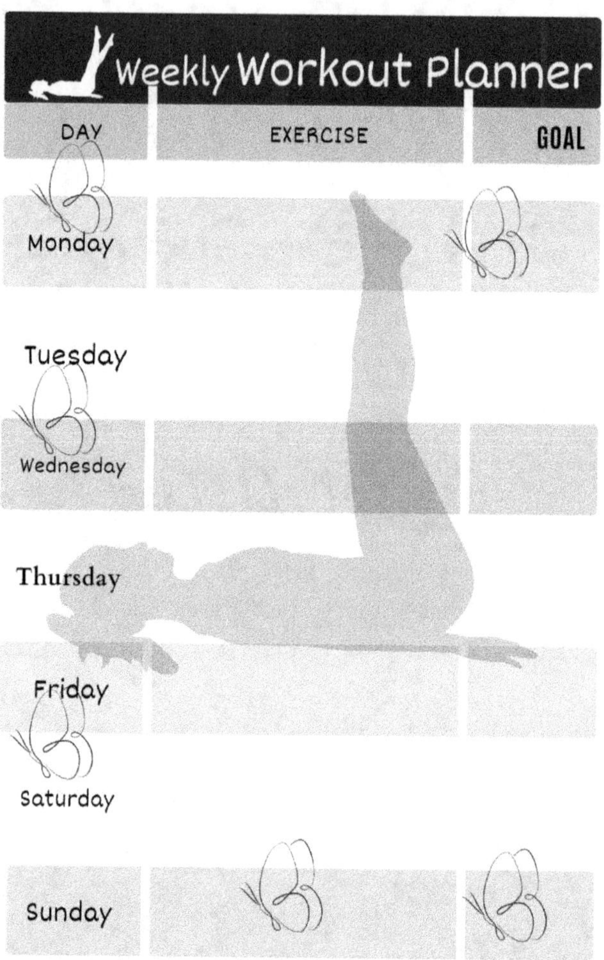

Weekly Workout Planner
DAY
EXERCISE
GOAL
Monday
Tuesday
Wednesday
Thursday
Friday
Saturday
Sunday

Weekly Workout Planner

DAY	EXERCISE	GOAL
Monday		
Tuesday		
Wednesday		
Thursday		
Friday		
Saturday		
Sunday		

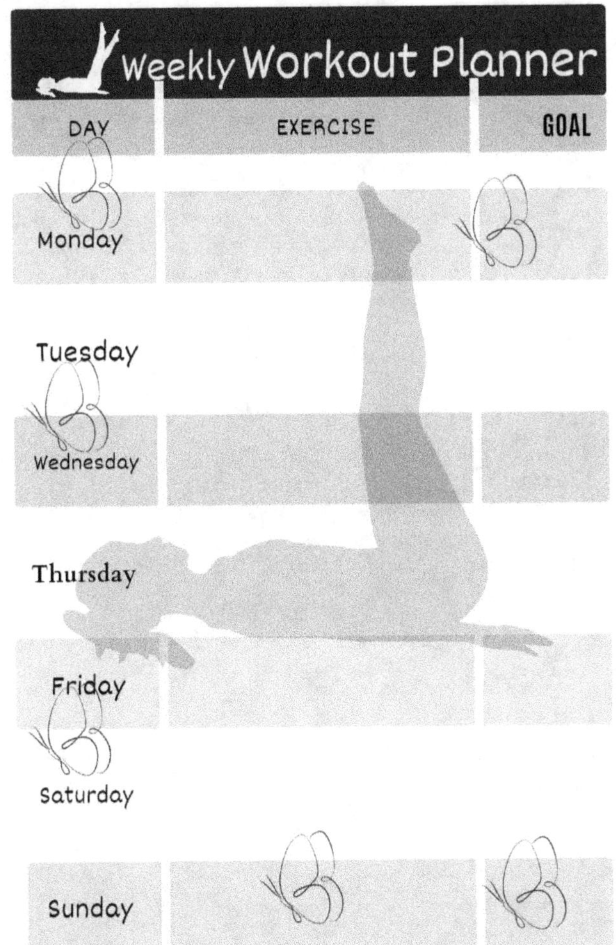

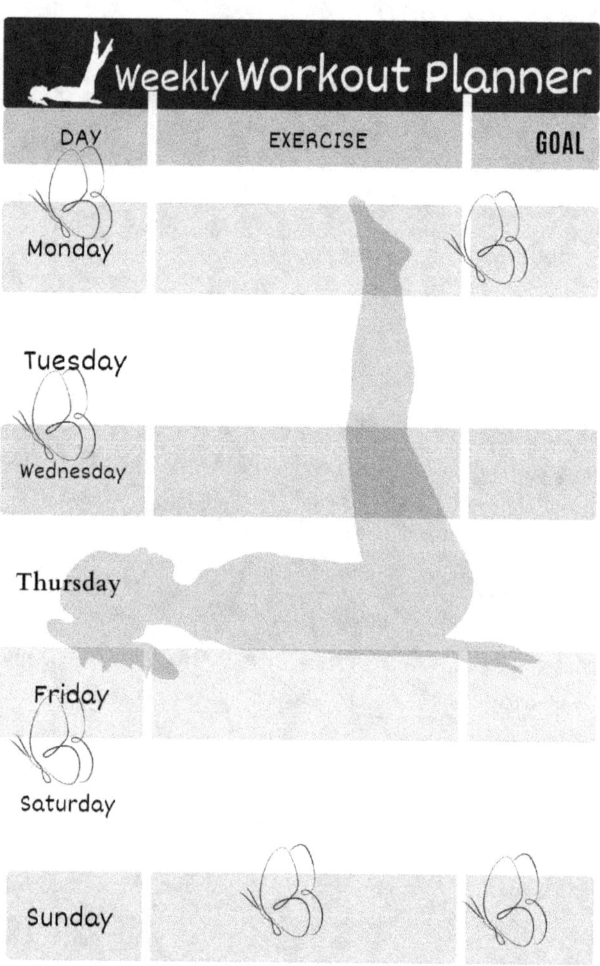
Weekly Workout Planner
DAY
EXERCISE
GOAL
Monday
Tuesday
Wednesday
Thursday
Friday
Saturday
Sunday

Weekly Workout Planner

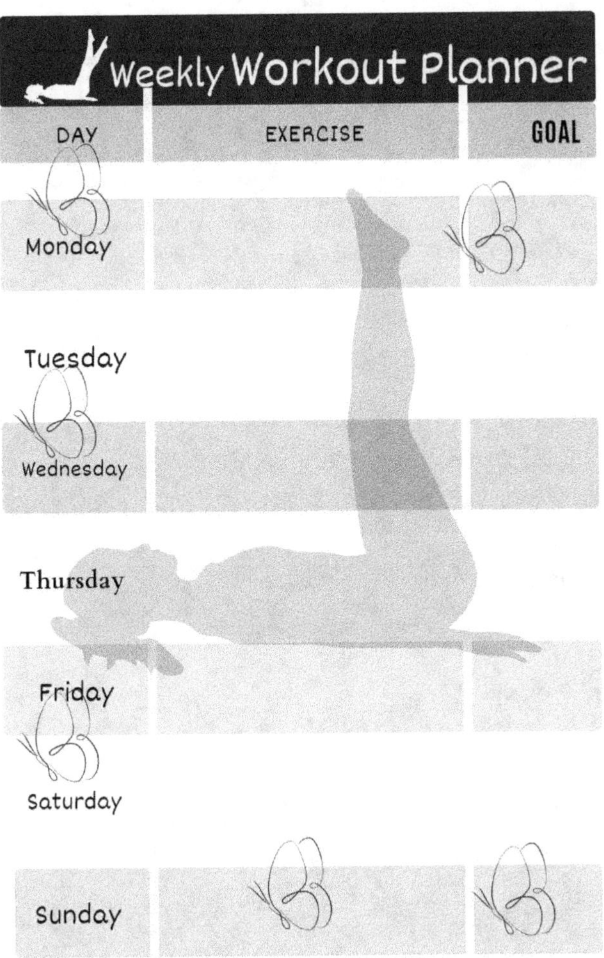

DAY	EXERCISE	GOAL
Monday		
Tuesday		
Wednesday		
Thursday		
Friday		
Saturday		
Sunday		

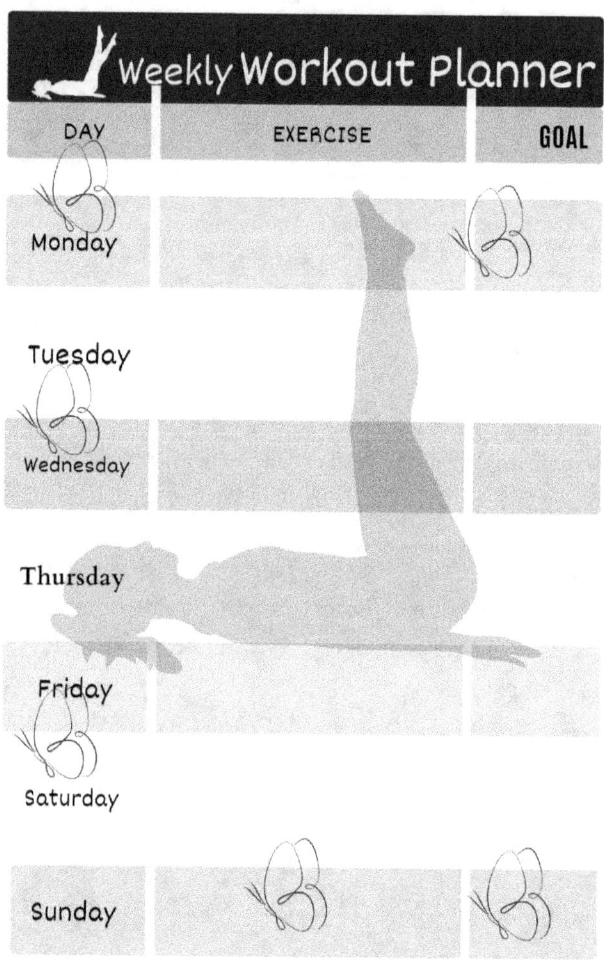
Weekly Workout Planner
DAY
EXERCISE
GOAL
Monday
Tuesday
Wednesday
Thursday
Friday
Saturday
Sunday

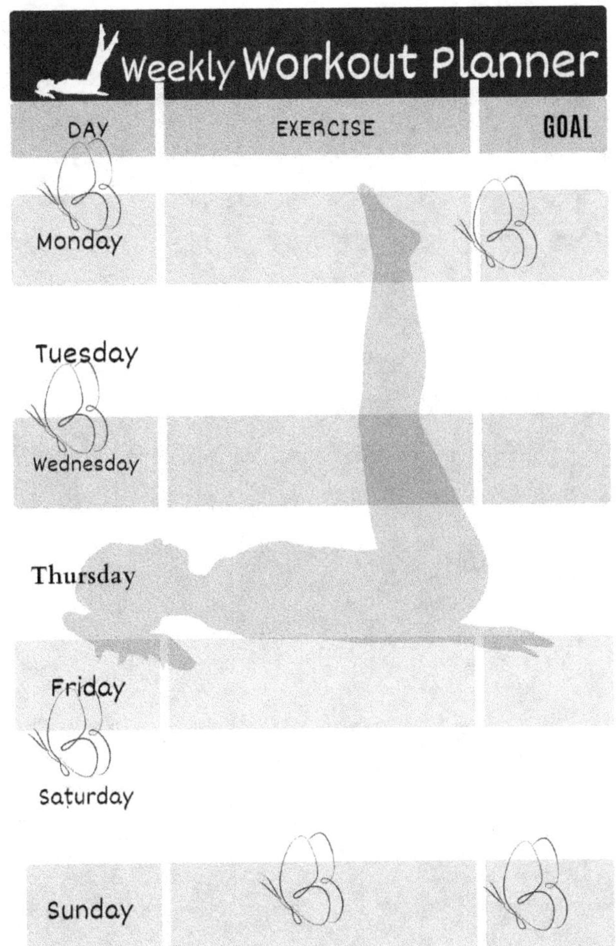

Weekly Workout Planner
DAY
EXERCISE
GOAL
Monday
Tuesday
Wednesday
Thursday
Friday
Saturday
Sunday

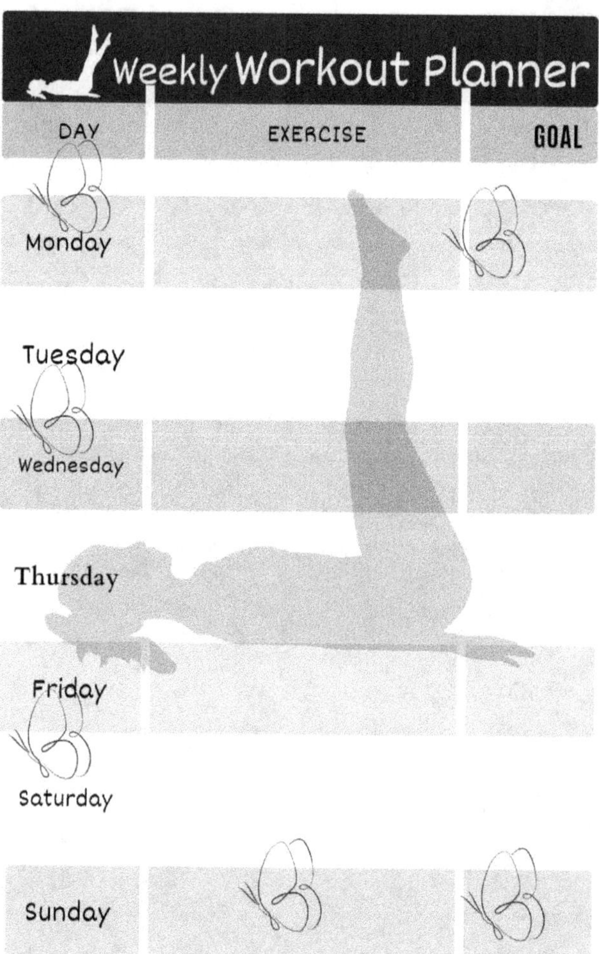

Weekly Workout Planner
DAY
EXERCISE
GOAL
Monday
Tuesday
Wednesday
Thursday
Friday
Saturday
Sunday

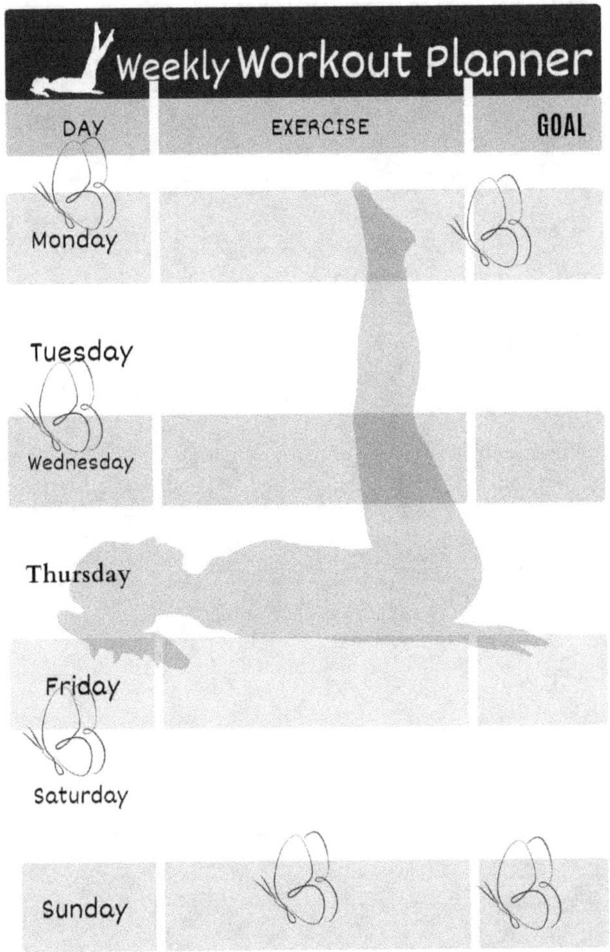

Weekly Workout Planner
DAY
EXERCISE
GOAL
Monday
Tuesday
Wednesday
Thursday
Friday
Saturday
Sunday

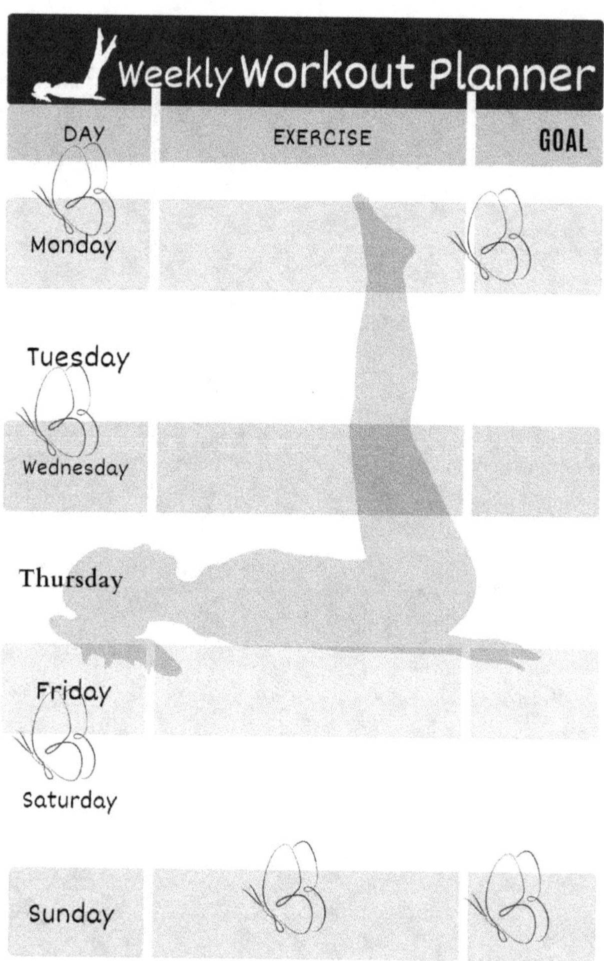

Weekly Workout Planner
DAY
EXERCISE
GOAL
Monday
Tuesday
Wednesday
Thursday
Friday
Saturday
Sunday

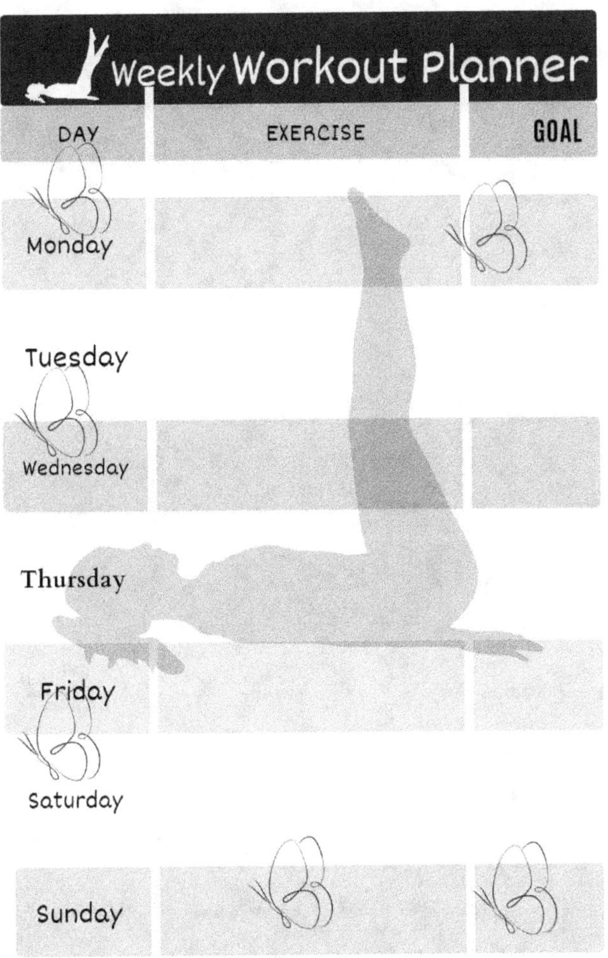

Weekly Workout Planner
DAY
EXERCISE
GOAL
Monday
Tuesday
Wednesday
Thursday
Friday
Saturday
Sunday

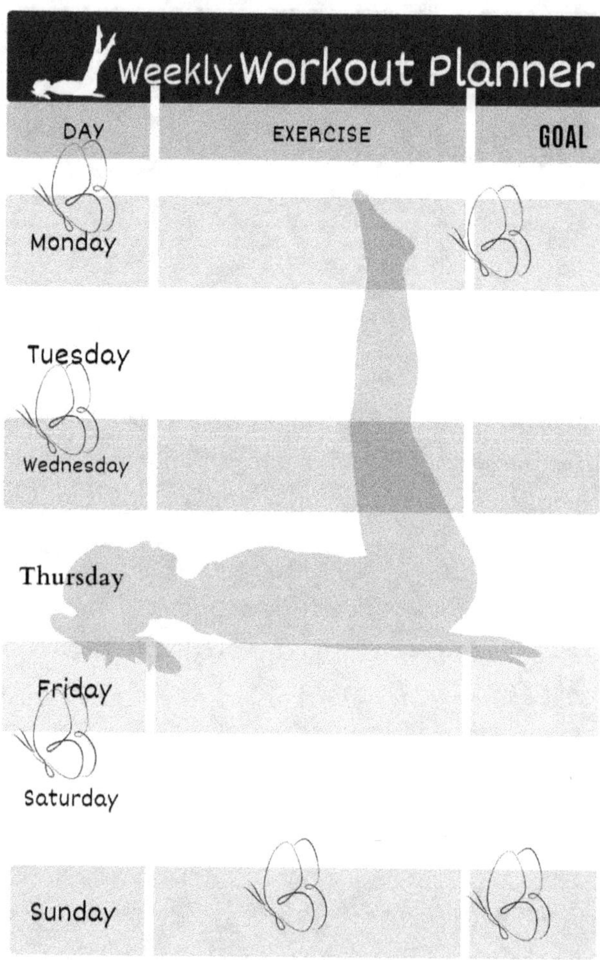

Weekly Workout Planner
DAY
EXERCISE
GOAL
Monday
Tuesday
Wednesday
Thursday
Friday
Saturday
Sunday

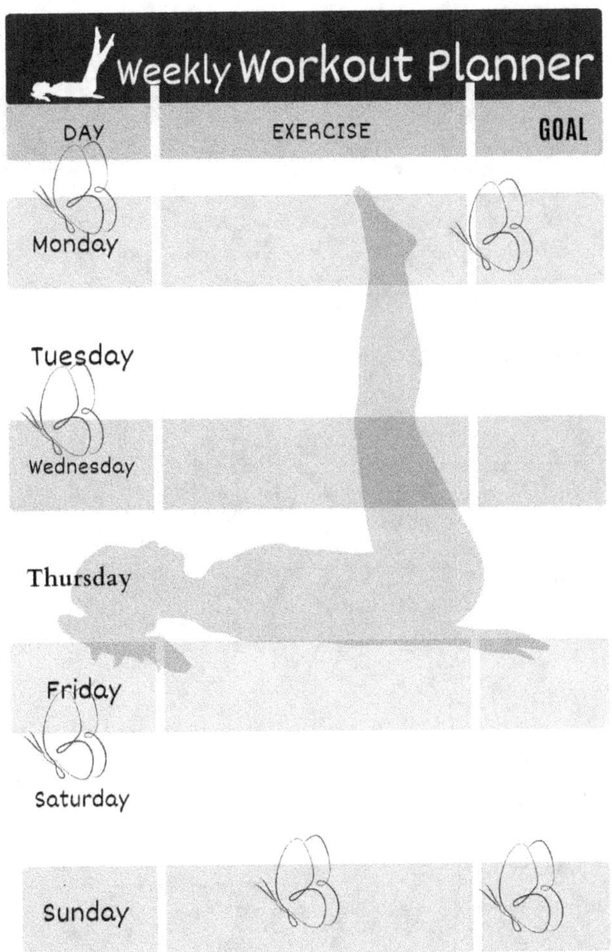
Weekly Workout Planner
DAY
EXERCISE
GOAL
Monday
Tuesday
Wednesday
Thursday
Friday
Saturday
Sunday

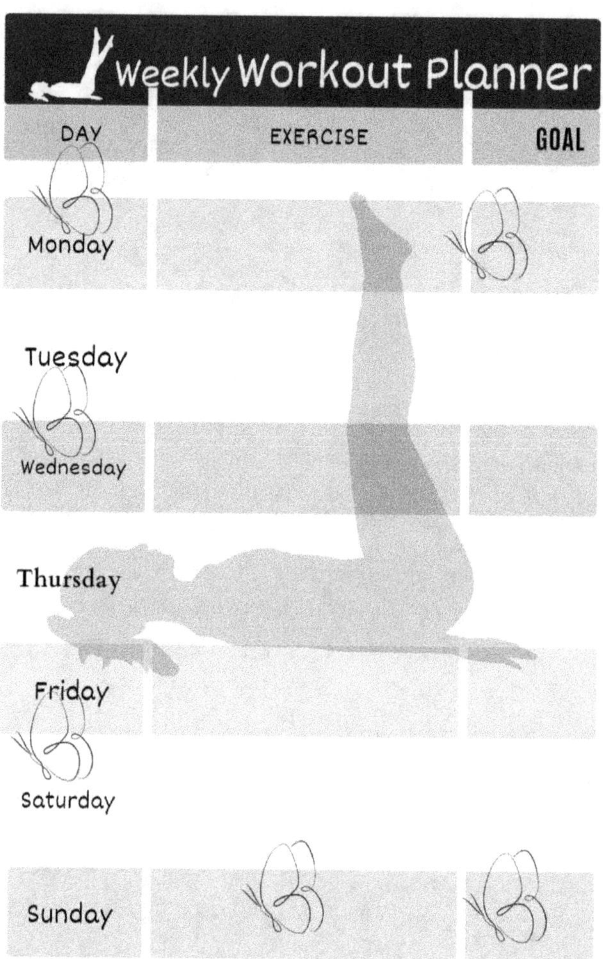

Weekly Workout Planner
DAY
EXERCISE
GOAL
Monday
Tuesday
Wednesday
Thursday
Friday
Saturday
Sunday

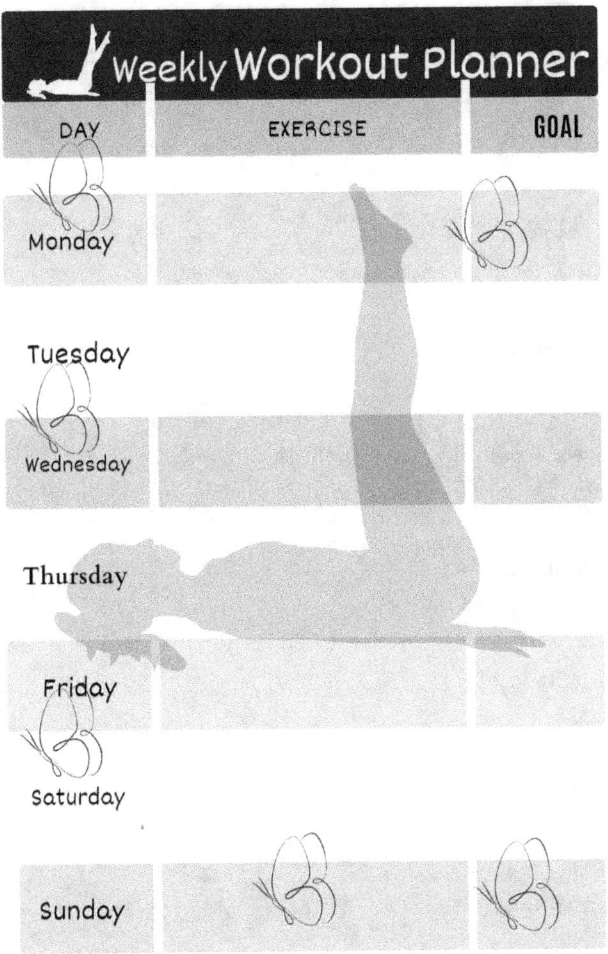

Weekly Workout Planner
DAY
EXERCISE
GOAL
Monday
Tuesday
Wednesday
Thursday
Friday
Saturday
Sunday

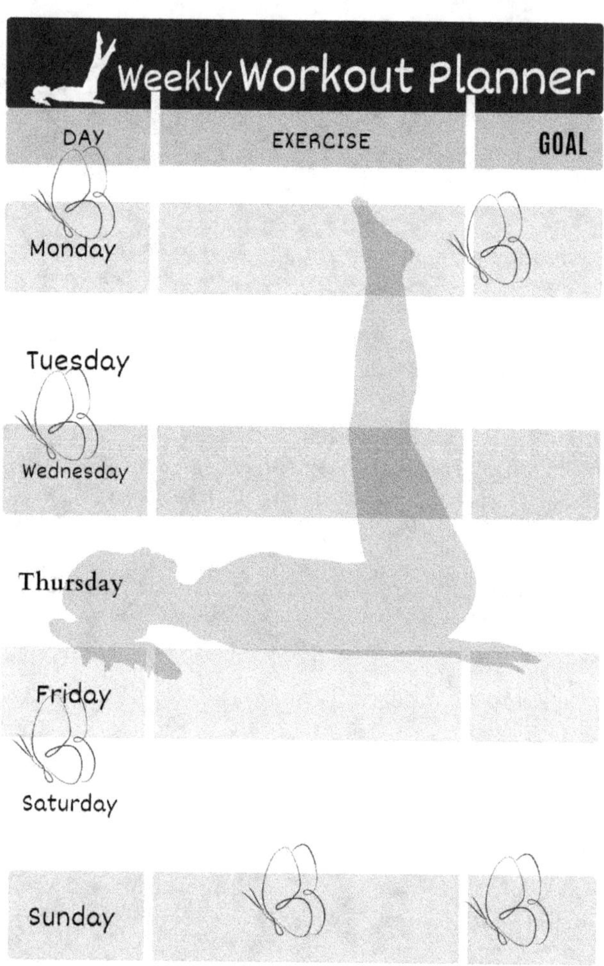
Weekly Workout Planner
DAY
EXERCISE
GOAL
Monday
Tuesday
Wednesday
Thursday
Friday
Saturday
Sunday

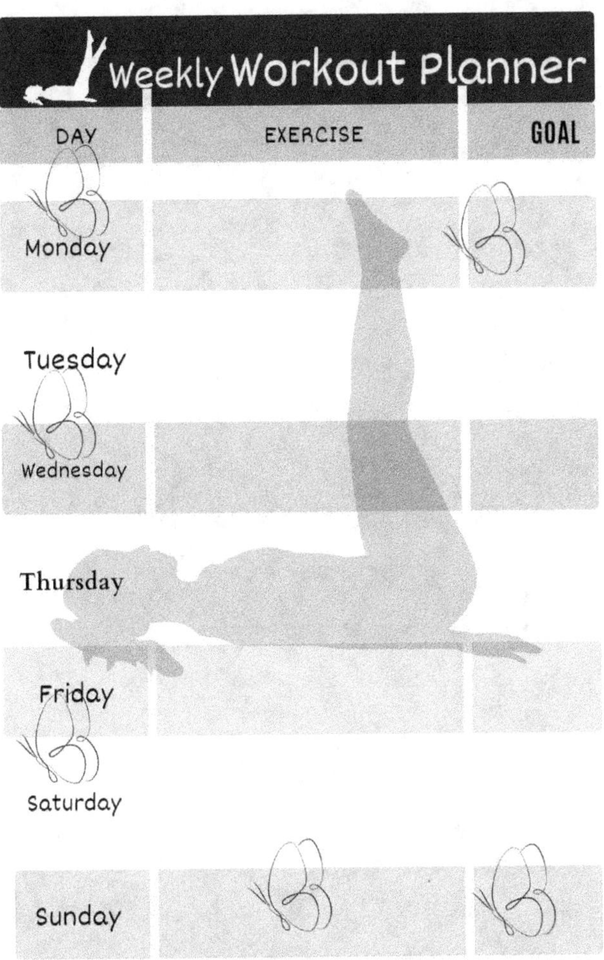

Weekly Workout Planner
DAY
EXERCISE
GOAL
Monday
Tuesday
Wednesday
Thursday
Friday
Saturday
Sunday

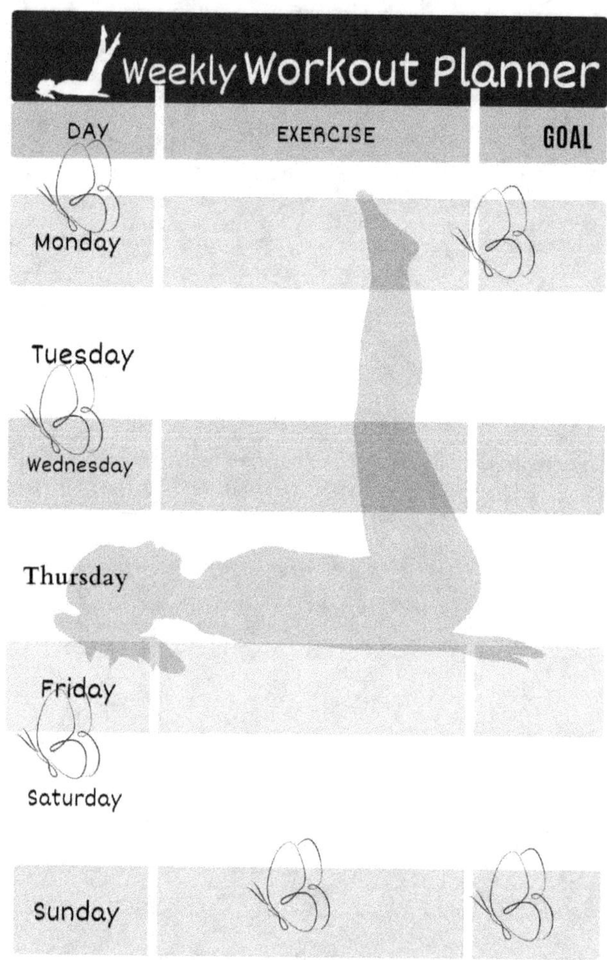

Weekly Workout Planner
DAY
EXERCISE
GOAL
Monday
Tuesday
Wednesday
Thursday
Friday
Saturday
Sunday

Weekly Workout Planner

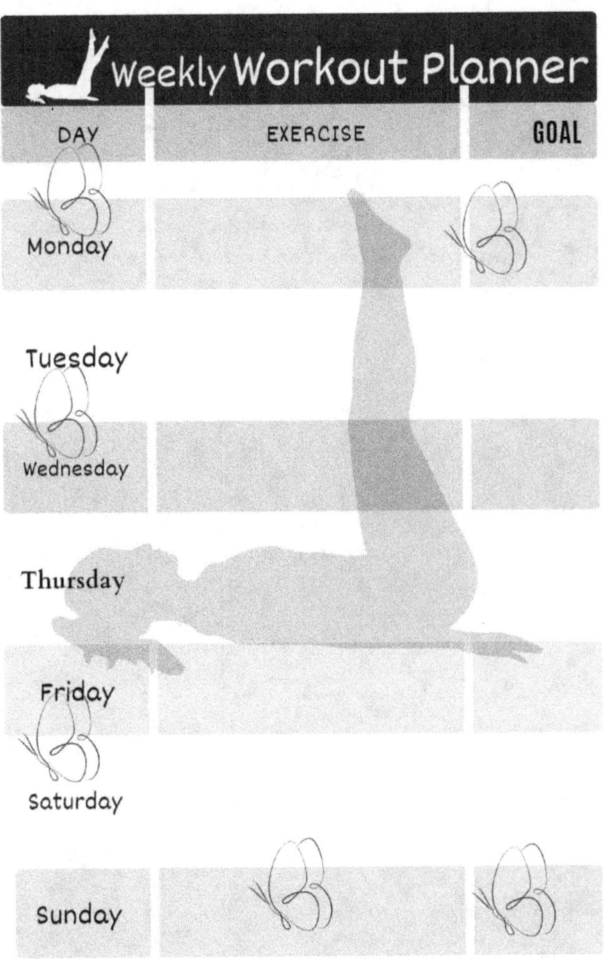

DAY	EXERCISE	GOAL
Monday		
Tuesday		
Wednesday		
Thursday		
Friday		
Saturday		
Sunday		

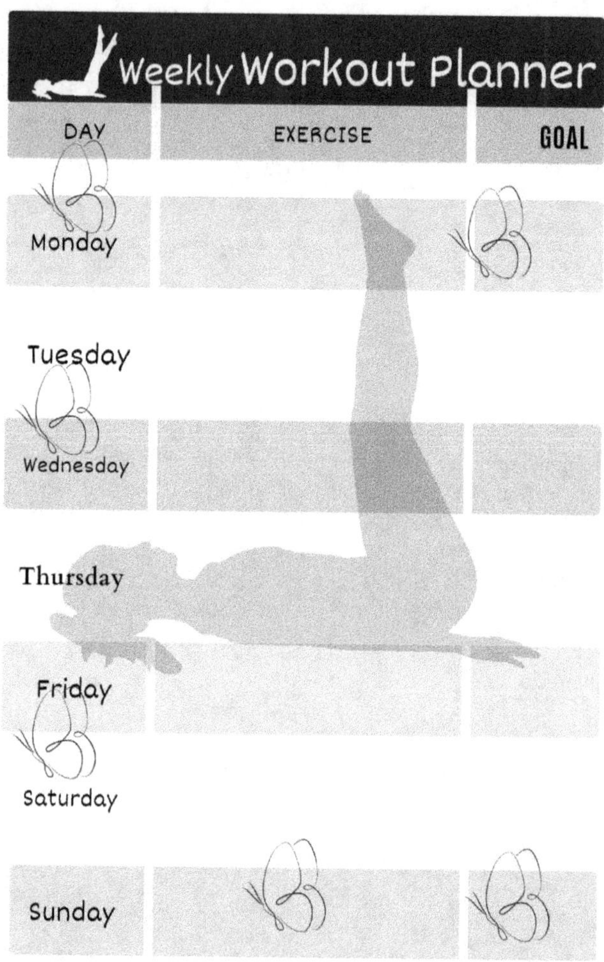
Weekly Workout Planner
DAY
EXERCISE
GOAL
Monday
Tuesday
Wednesday
Thursday
Friday
Saturday
Sunday

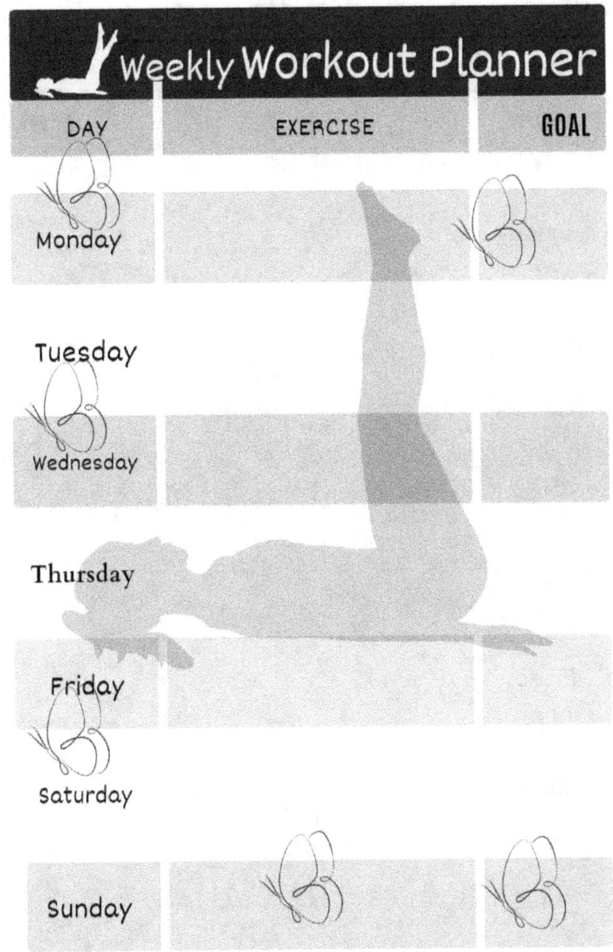

Weekly Workout Planner
DAY
EXERCISE
GOAL
Monday
Tuesday
Wednesday
Thursday
Friday
Saturday
Sunday

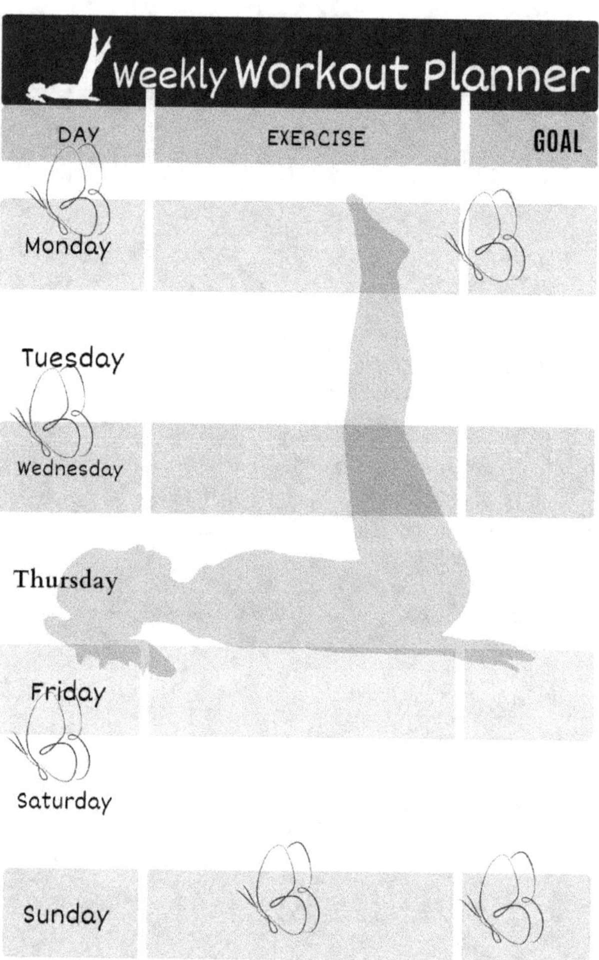

Weekly Workout Planner
DAY
EXERCISE
GOAL
Monday
Tuesday
Wednesday
Thursday
Friday
Saturday
Sunday

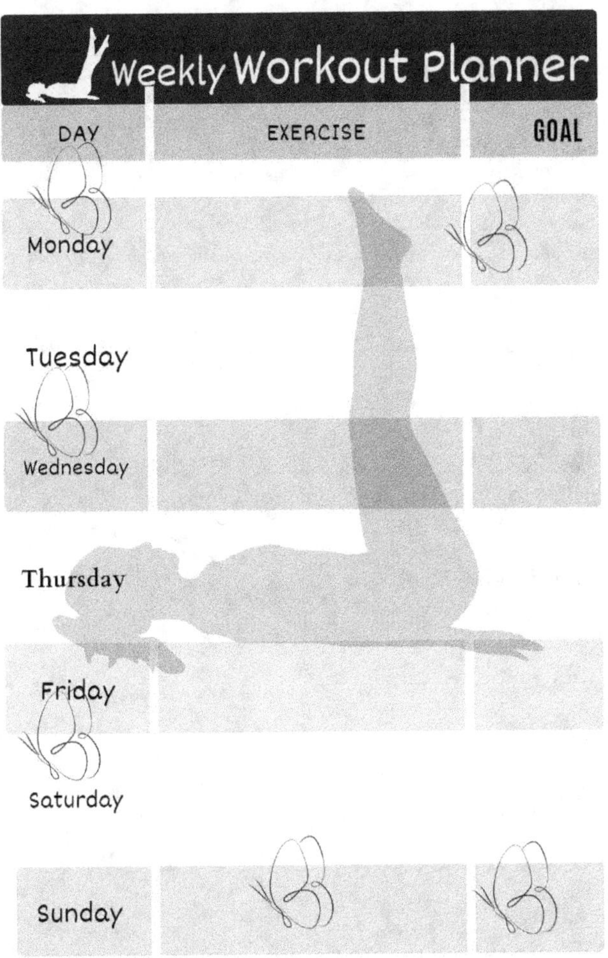

Weekly Workout Planner
DAY
EXERCISE
GOAL
Monday
Tuesday
Wednesday
Thursday
Friday
Saturday
Sunday

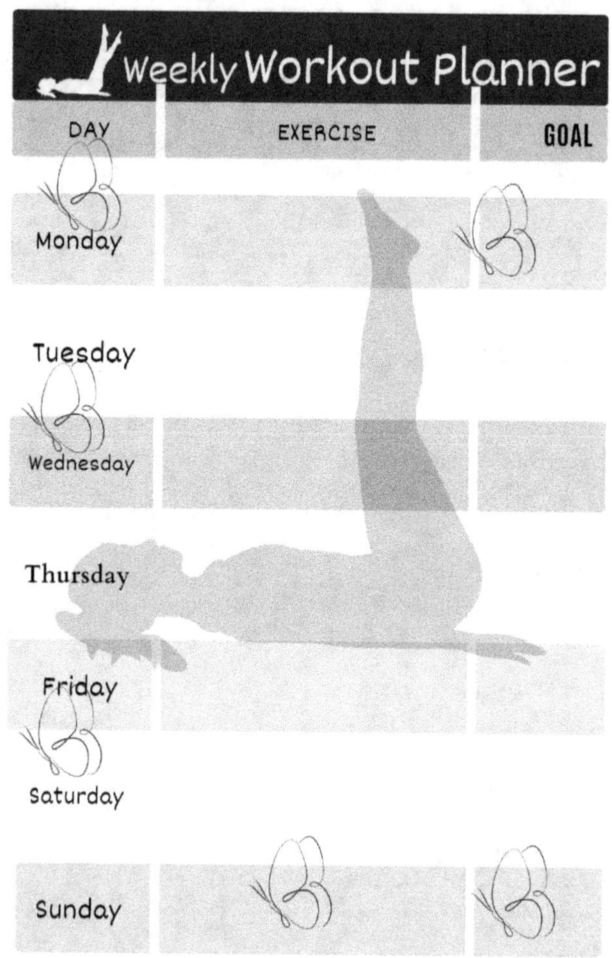

Weekly Workout Planner
DAY
EXERCISE
GOAL
Monday
Tuesday
Wednesday
Thursday
Friday
Saturday
Sunday

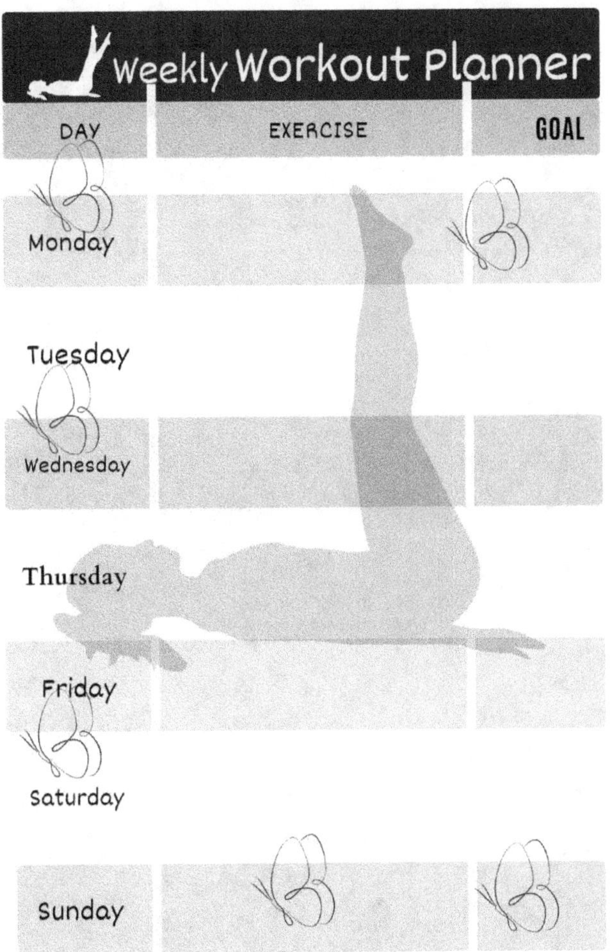

Weekly Workout Planner
DAY
EXERCISE
GOAL
Monday
Tuesday
Wednesday
Thursday
Friday
Saturday
Sunday

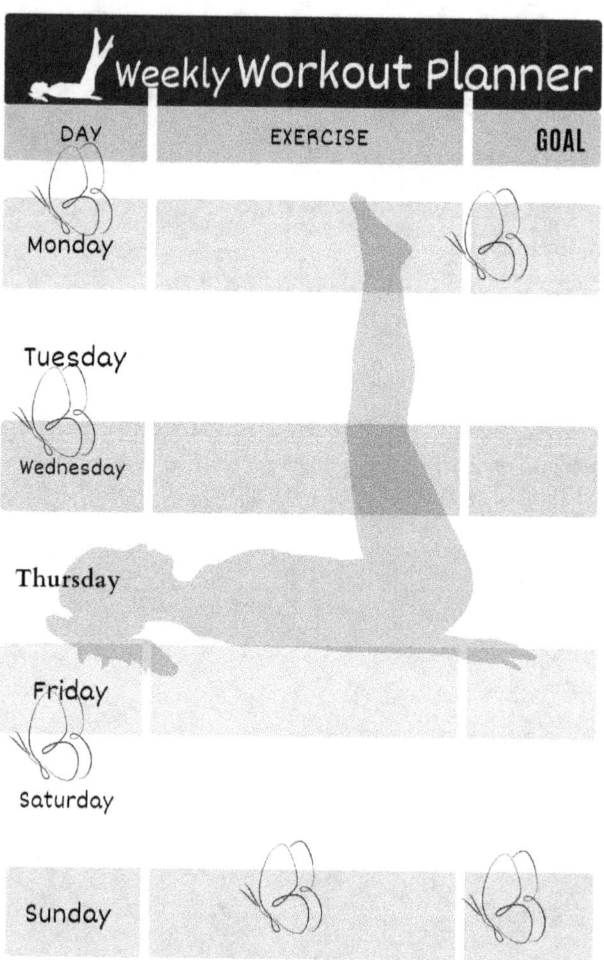

Weekly Workout Planner
DAY
EXERCISE
GOAL
Monday
Tuesday
Wednesday
Thursday
Friday
Saturday
Sunday

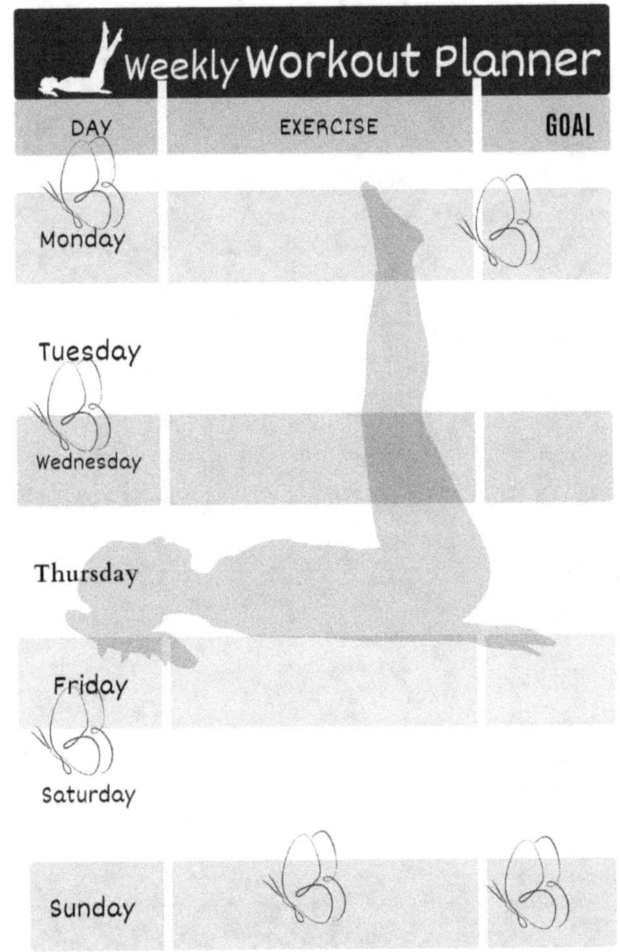

Weekly Workout Planner
DAY
EXERCISE
GOAL
Monday
Tuesday
Wednesday
Thursday
Friday
Saturday
Sunday

Weekly Workout Planner

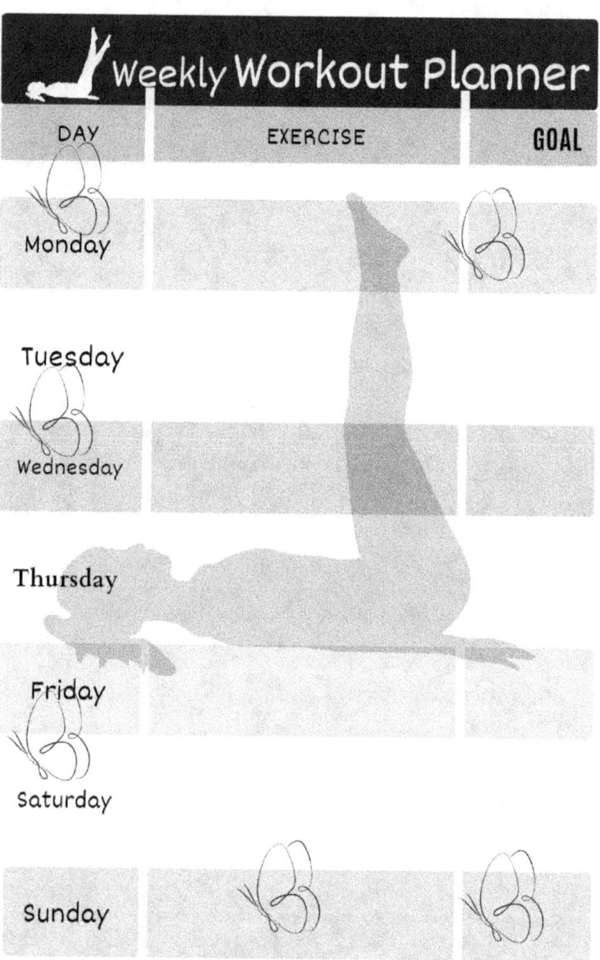

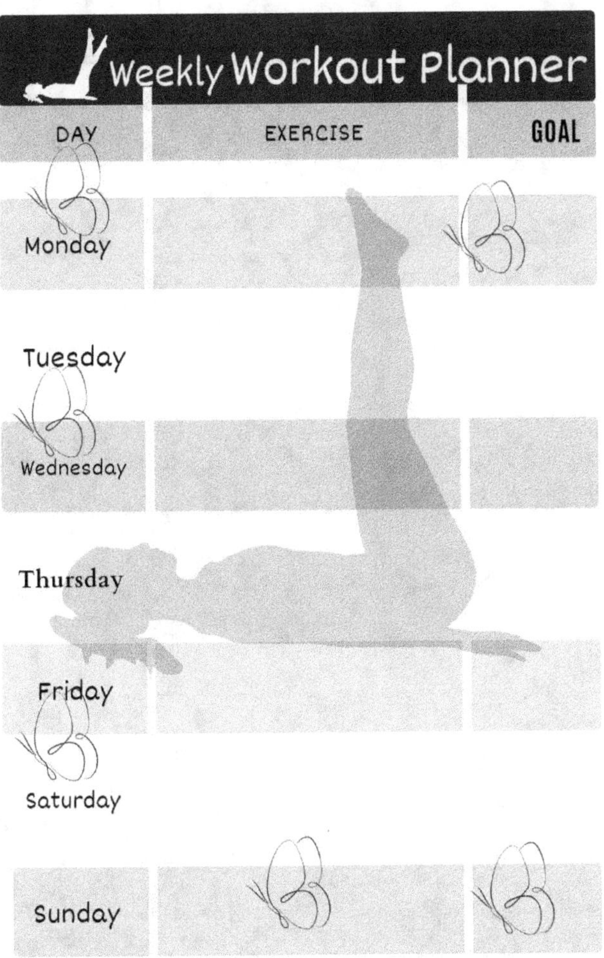

Weekly Workout Planner

DAY	EXERCISE	GOAL
Monday		
Tuesday		
Wednesday		
Thursday		
Friday		
Saturday		
Sunday		

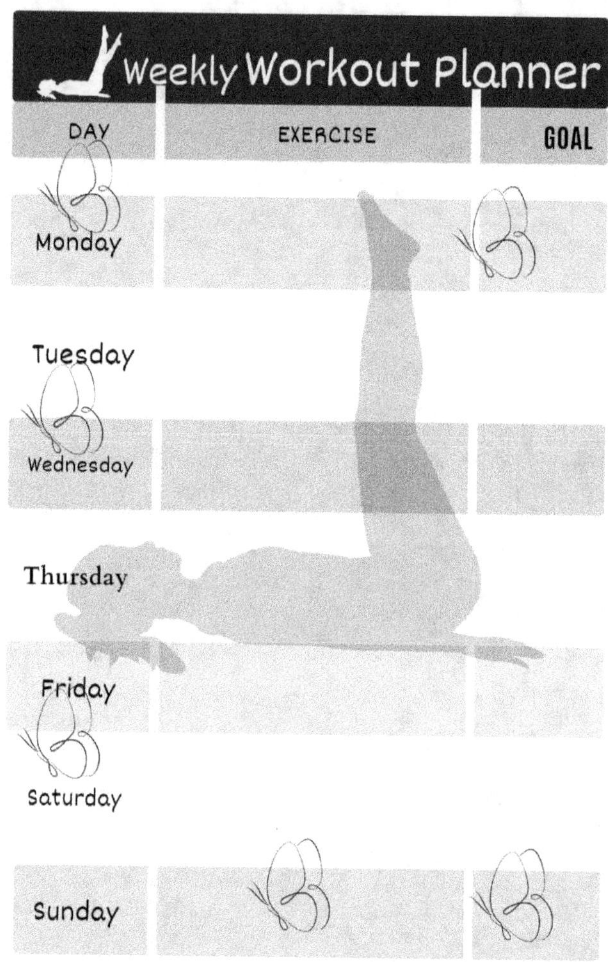
Weekly Workout Planner
DAY
EXERCISE
GOAL
Monday
Tuesday
Wednesday
Thursday
Friday
Saturday
Sunday

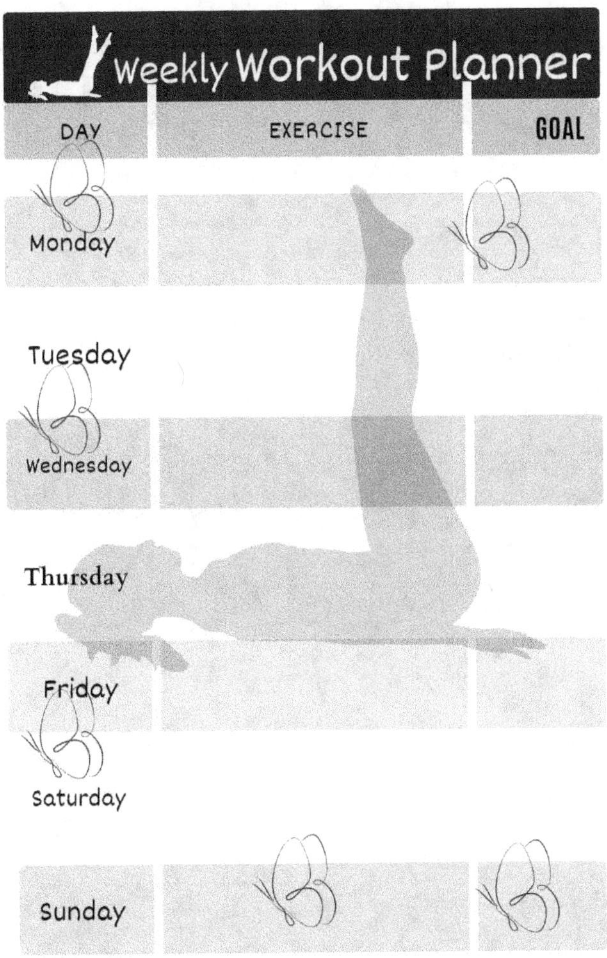
Weekly Workout Planner
DAY
EXERCISE
GOAL
Monday
Tuesday
Wednesday
Thursday
Friday
Saturday
Sunday

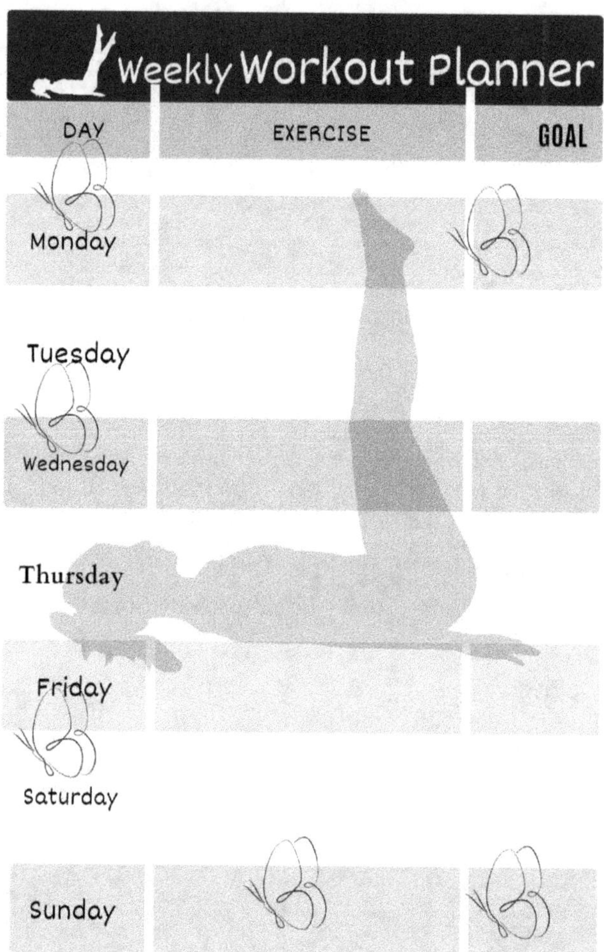

Weekly Workout Planner
DAY
EXERCISE
GOAL
Monday
Tuesday
Wednesday
Thursday
Friday
Saturday
Sunday

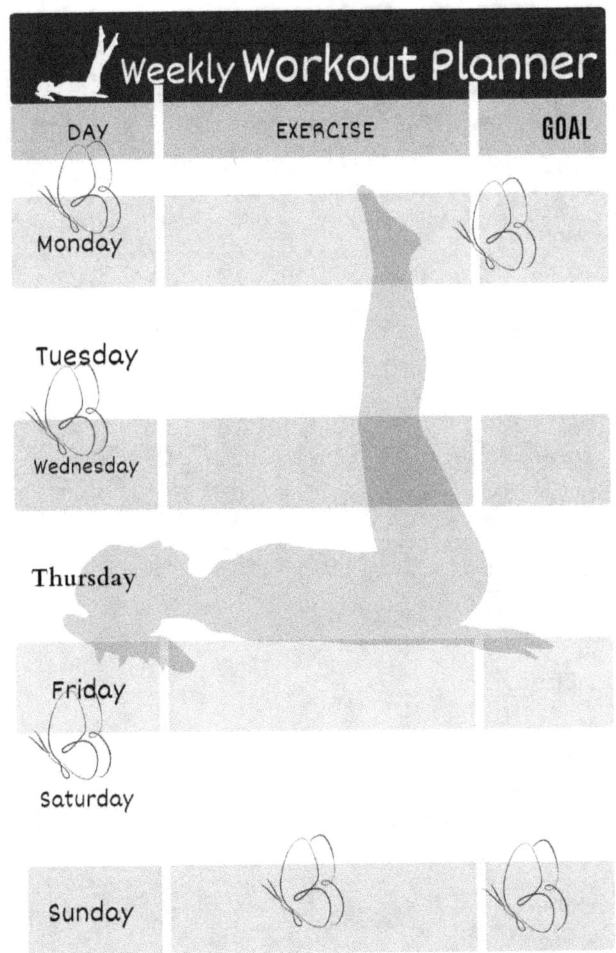

Weekly Workout Planner
DAY
EXERCISE
GOAL
Monday
Tuesday
Wednesday
Thursday
Friday
Saturday
Sunday

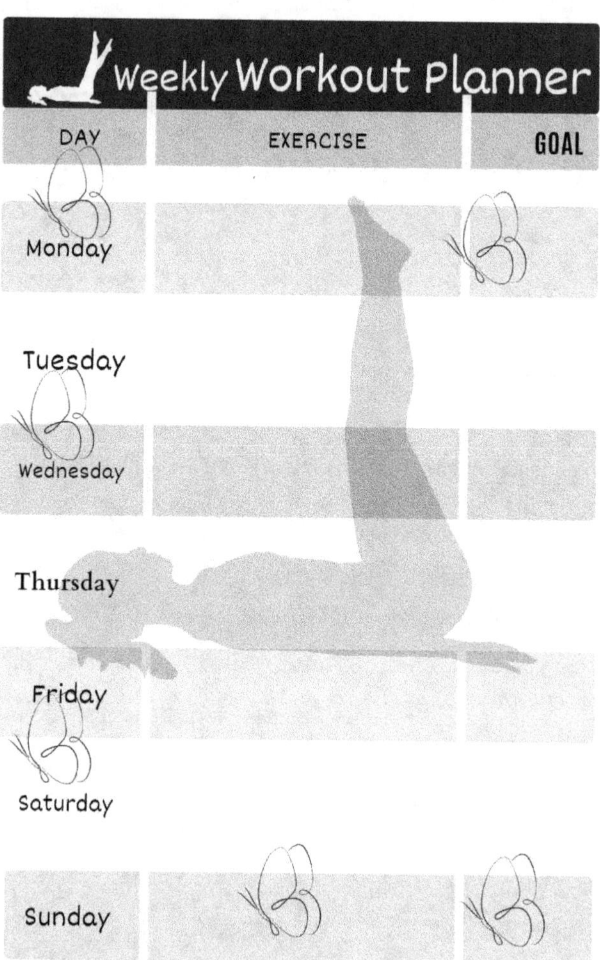

Weekly Workout Planner
DAY
EXERCISE
GOAL
Monday
Tuesday
Wednesday
Thursday
Friday
Saturday
Sunday

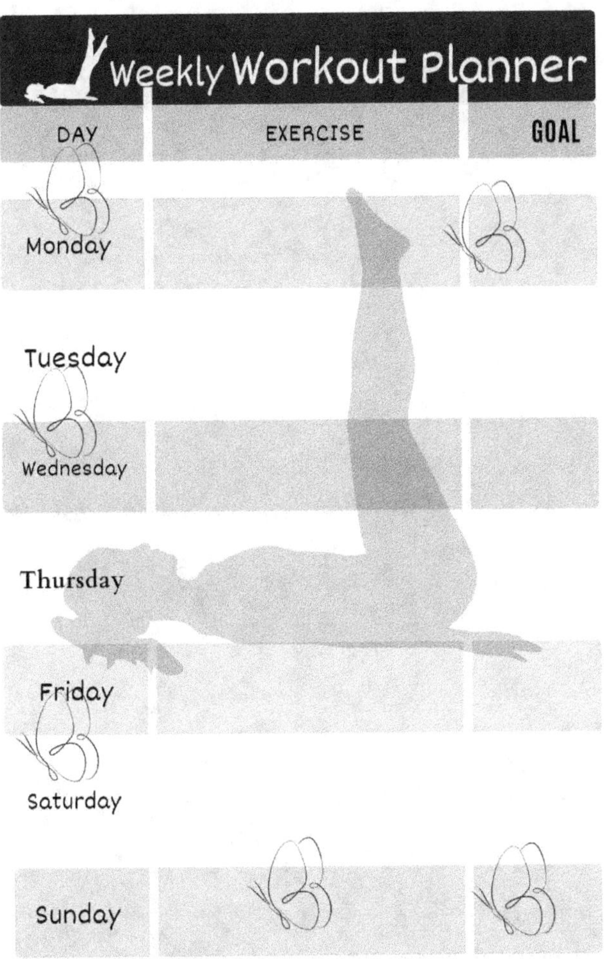

Weekly Workout Planner
DAY
EXERCISE
GOAL
Monday
Tuesday
Wednesday
Thursday
Friday
Saturday
Sunday

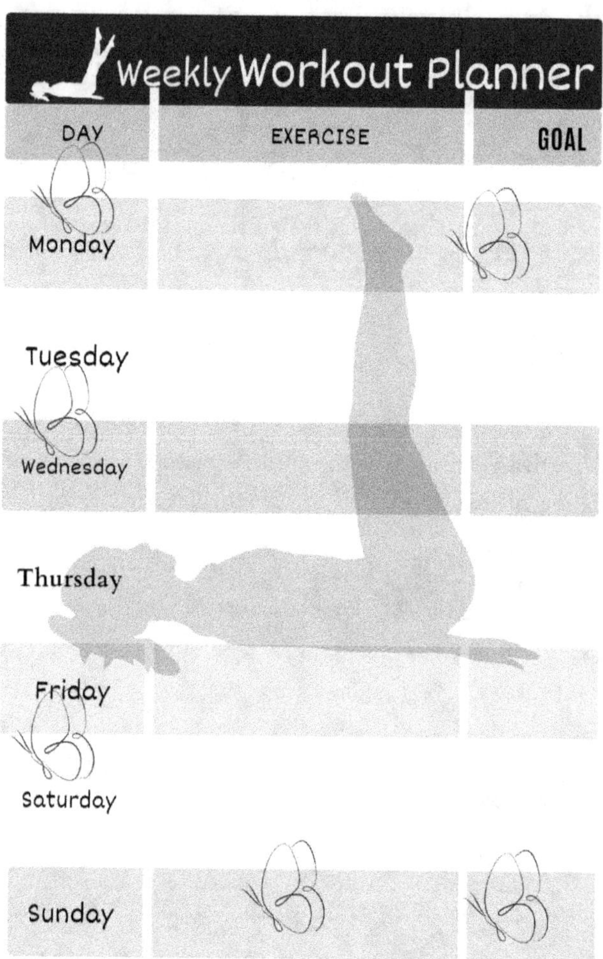

Weekly Workout Planner
DAY
EXERCISE
GOAL
Monday
Tuesday
Wednesday
Thursday
Friday
Saturday
Sunday

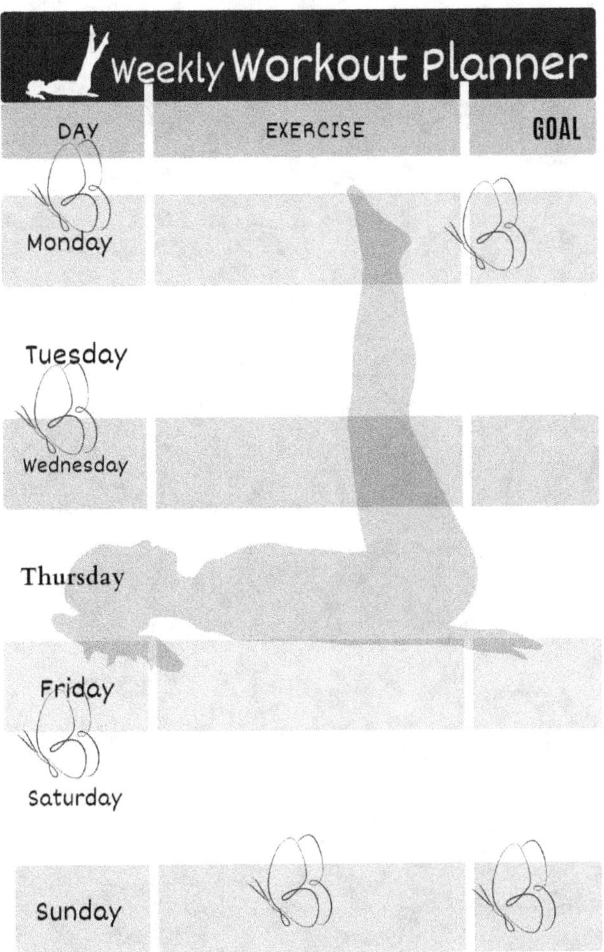

Weekly Workout Planner
DAY
EXERCISE
GOAL
Monday
Tuesday
Wednesday
Thursday
Friday
Saturday
Sunday

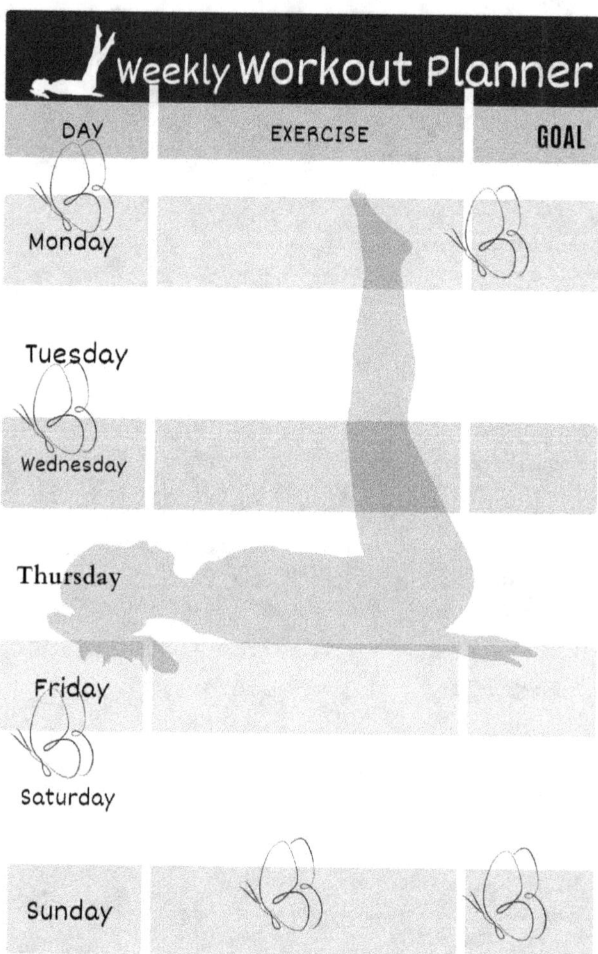

Weekly Workout Planner
DAY
EXERCISE
GOAL
Monday
Tuesday
Wednesday
Thursday
Friday
Saturday
Sunday

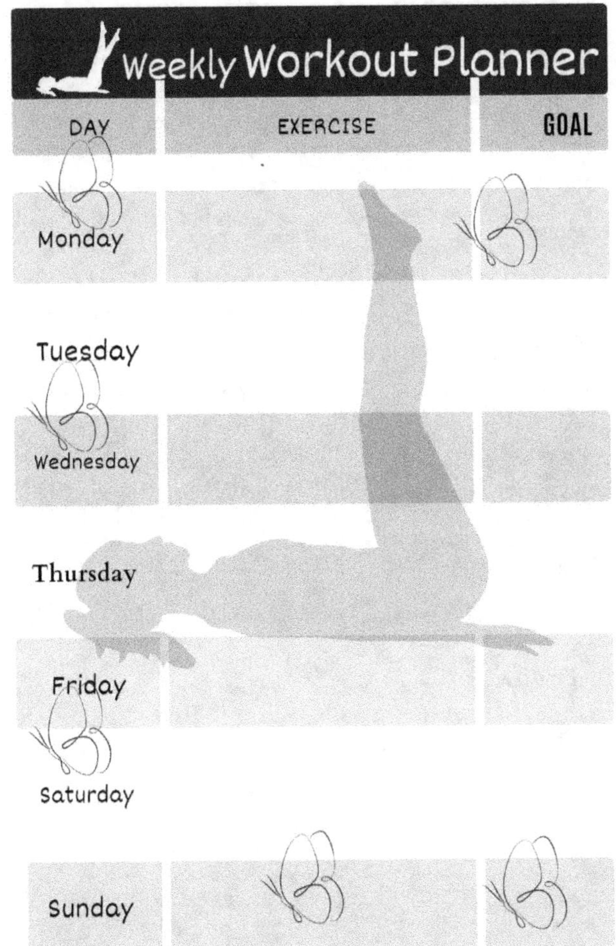

Weekly Workout Planner
DAY
EXERCISE
GOAL
Monday
Tuesday
Wednesday
Thursday
Friday
Saturday
Sunday

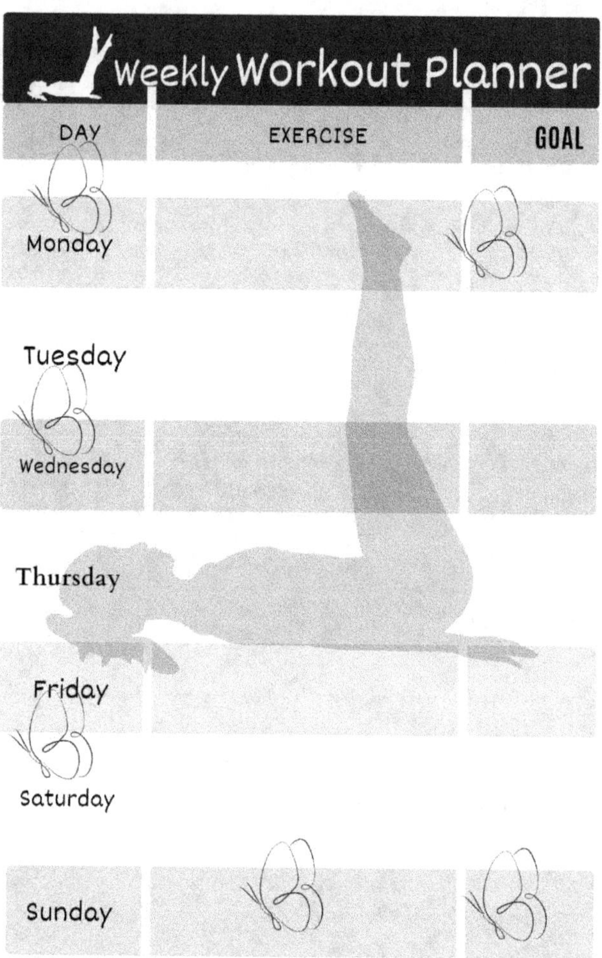

Weekly Workout Planner
DAY
EXERCISE
GOAL
Monday
Tuesday
Wednesday
Thursday
Friday
Saturday
Sunday

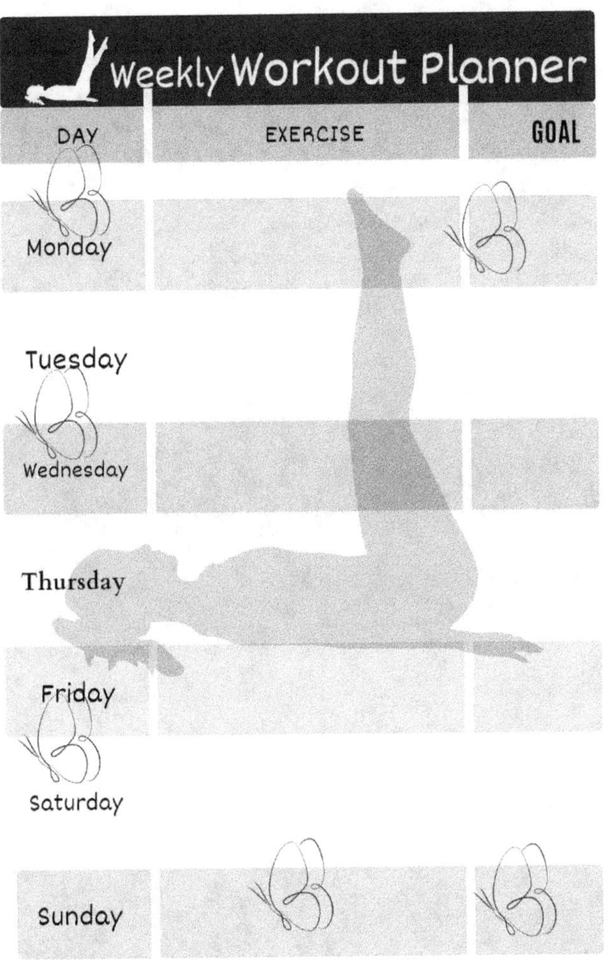

Weekly Workout Planner
DAY
EXERCISE
GOAL
Monday
Tuesday
Wednesday
Thursday
Friday
Saturday
Sunday

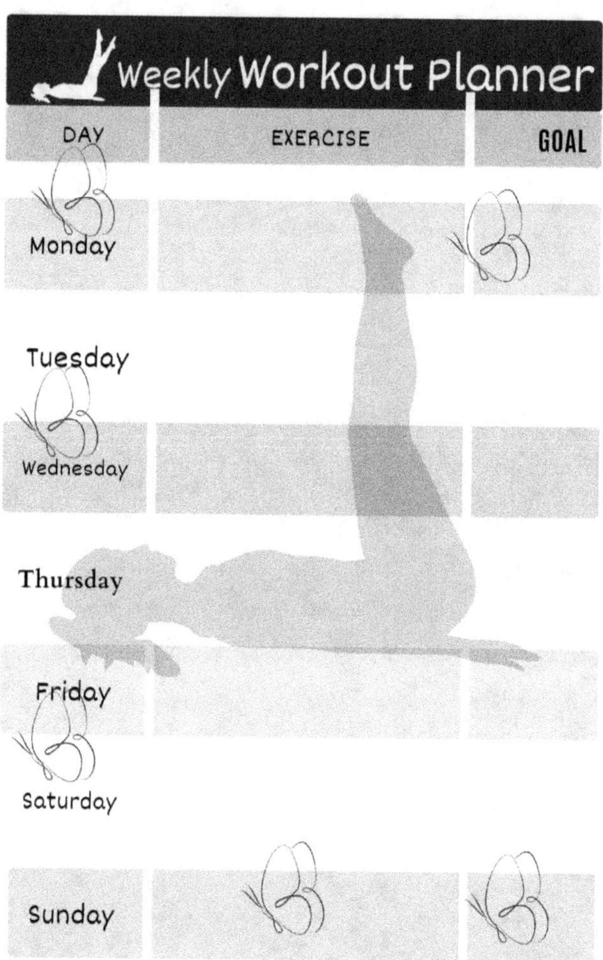

Weekly Workout Planner
DAY
EXERCISE
GOAL
Monday
Tuesday
Wednesday
Thursday
Friday
Saturday
Sunday

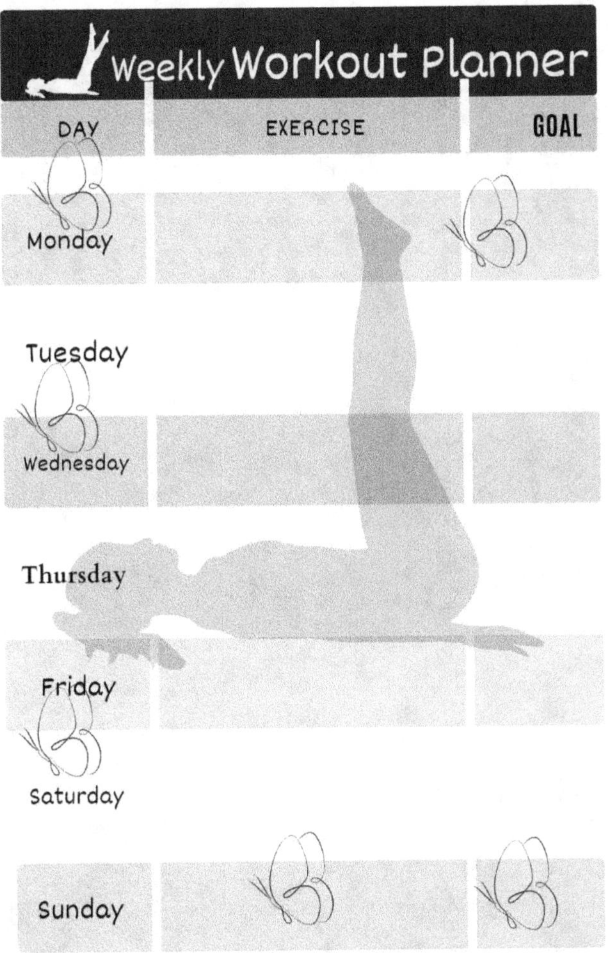

Weekly Workout Planner
DAY
EXERCISE
GOAL
Monday
Tuesday
Wednesday
Thursday
Friday
Saturday
Sunday

Weekly Workout Planner

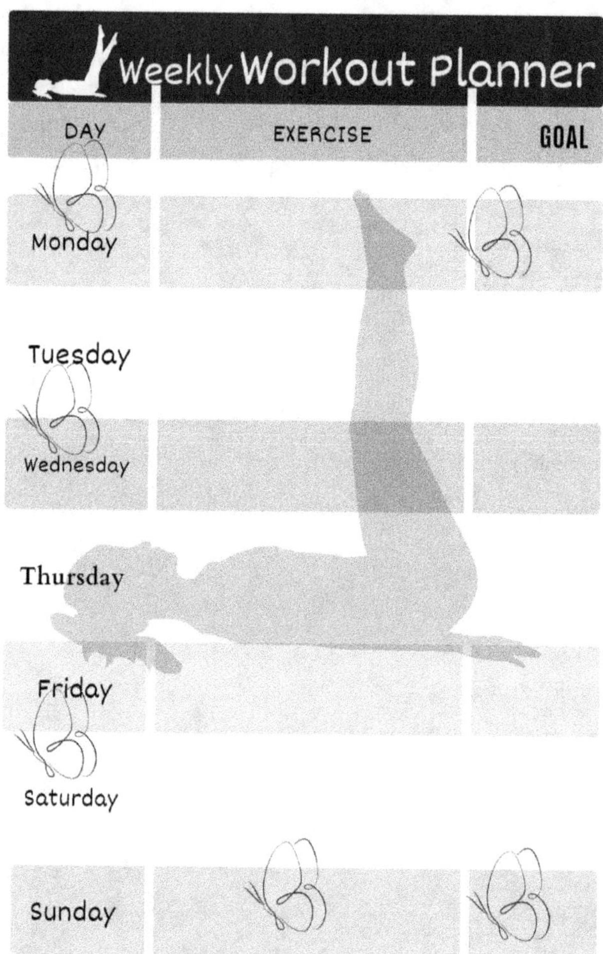

DAY	EXERCISE	GOAL
Monday		
Tuesday		
Wednesday		
Thursday		
Friday		
Saturday		
Sunday		

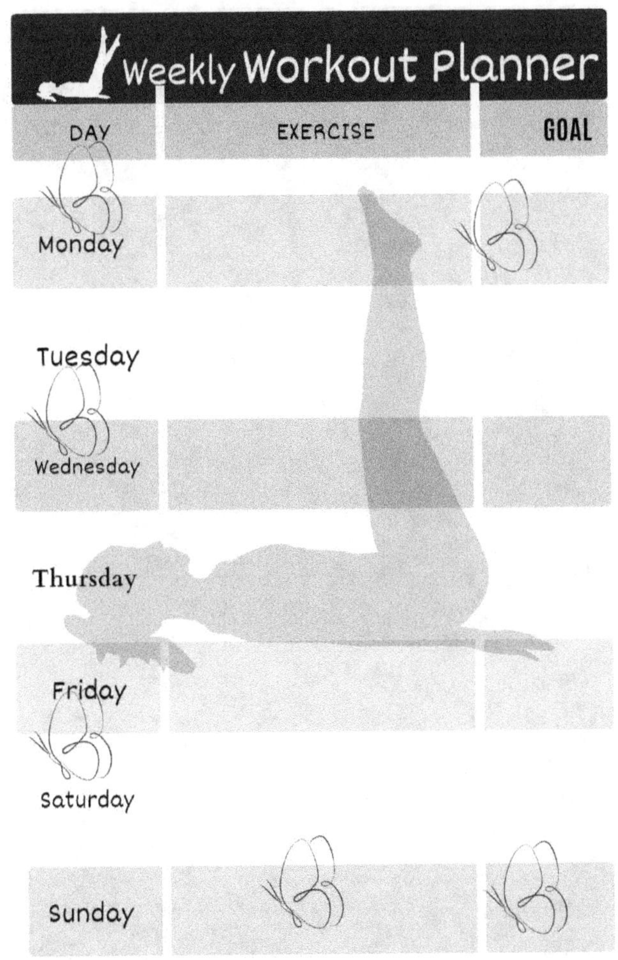

Weekly Workout Planner
DAY
EXERCISE
GOAL
Monday
Tuesday
Wednesday
Thursday
Friday
Saturday
Sunday

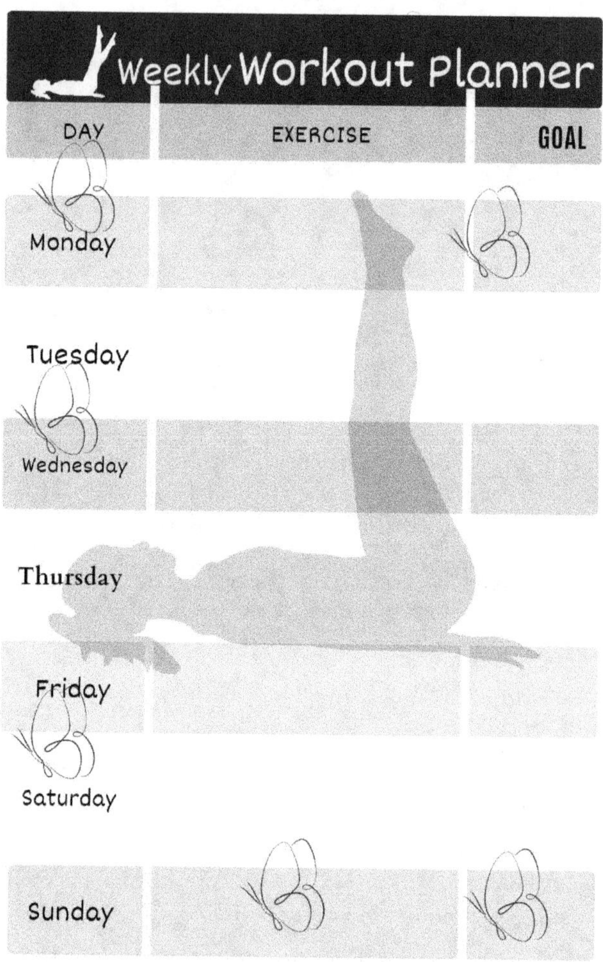

Weekly Workout Planner
DAY
EXERCISE
GOAL
Monday
Tuesday
Wednesday
Thursday
Friday
Saturday
Sunday

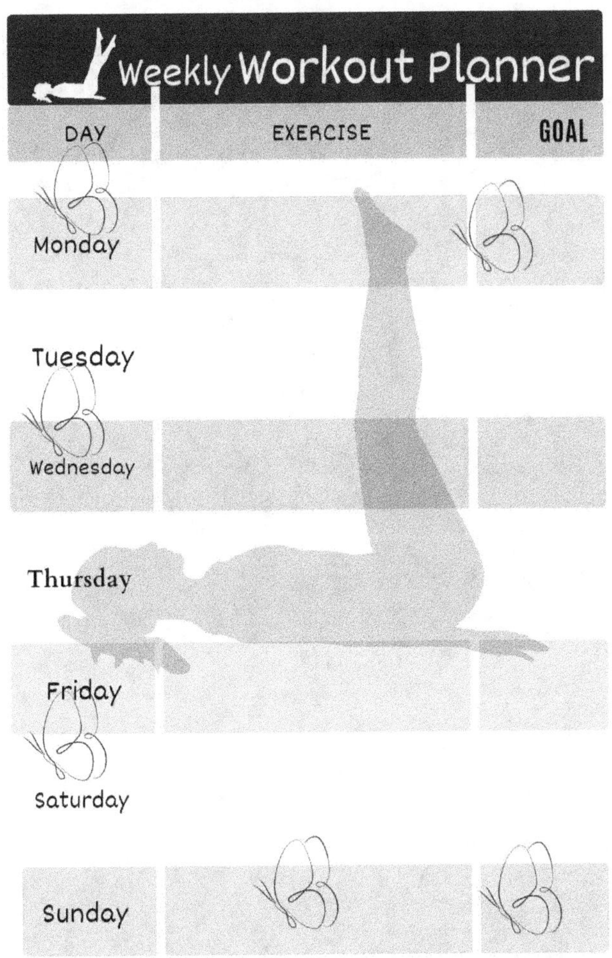

194

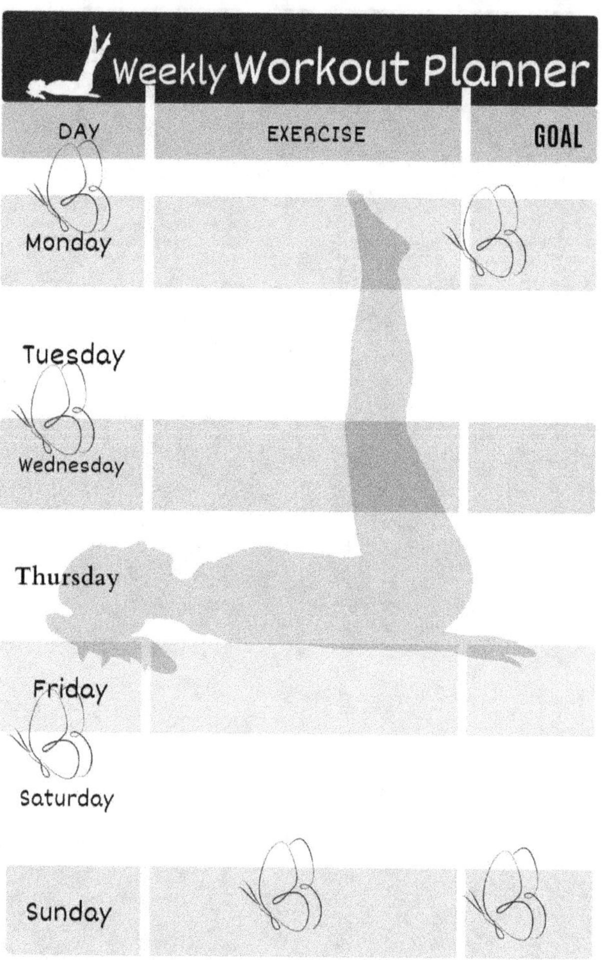

Weekly Workout Planner
DAY
EXERCISE
GOAL
Monday
Tuesday
Wednesday
Thursday
Friday
Saturday
Sunday

Weekly Workout Planner

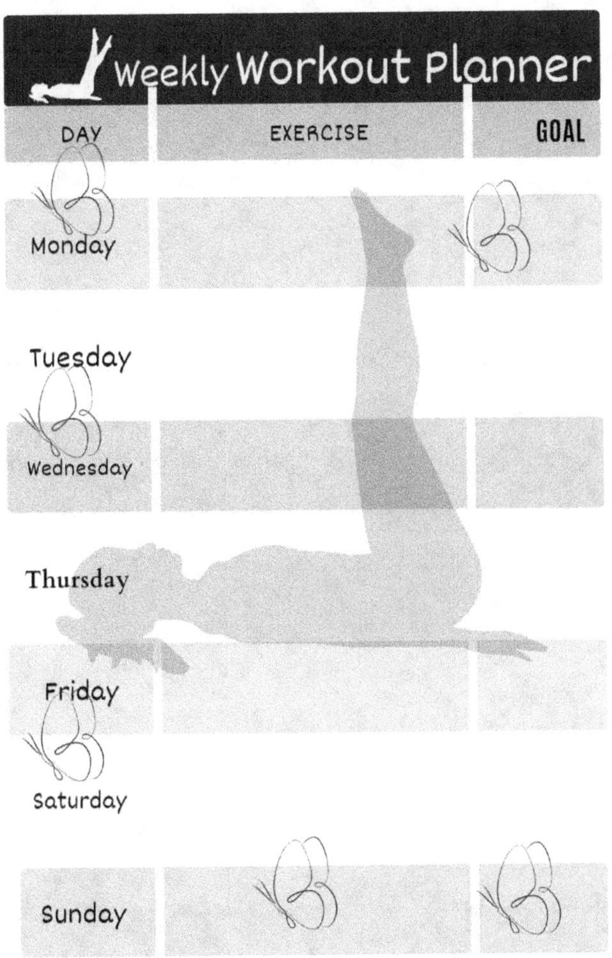

DAY	EXERCISE	GOAL
Monday		
Tuesday		
Wednesday		
Thursday		
Friday		
Saturday		
Sunday		

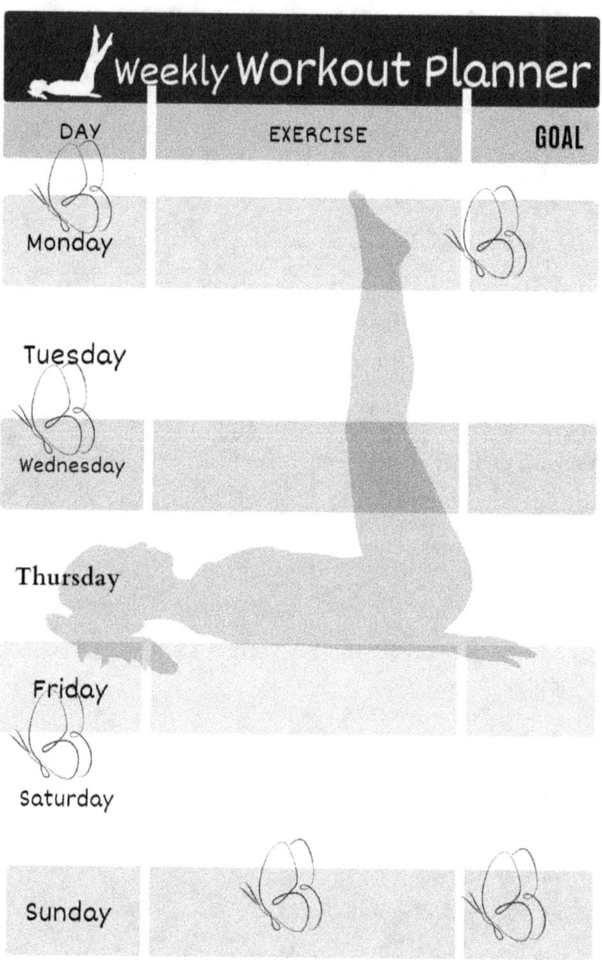
Weekly Workout Planner
DAY
EXERCISE
GOAL
Monday
Tuesday
Wednesday
Thursday
Friday
Saturday
Sunday

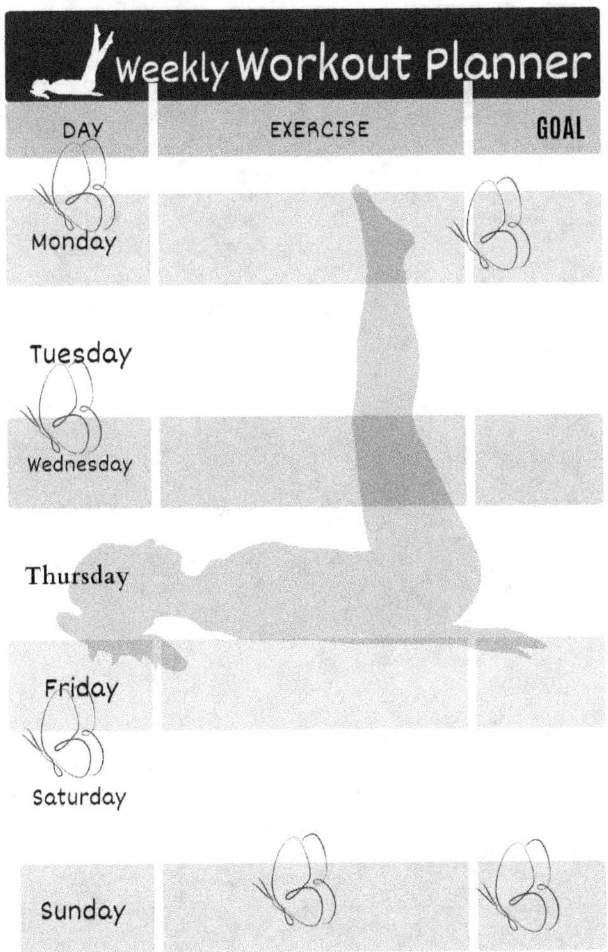

Weekly Workout Planner
DAY
EXERCISE
GOAL
Monday
Tuesday
Wednesday
Thursday
Friday
Saturday
Sunday

Weekly Workout Planner

DAY	EXERCISE	GOAL
Monday		
Tuesday		
Wednesday		
Thursday		
Friday		
Saturday		
Sunday		

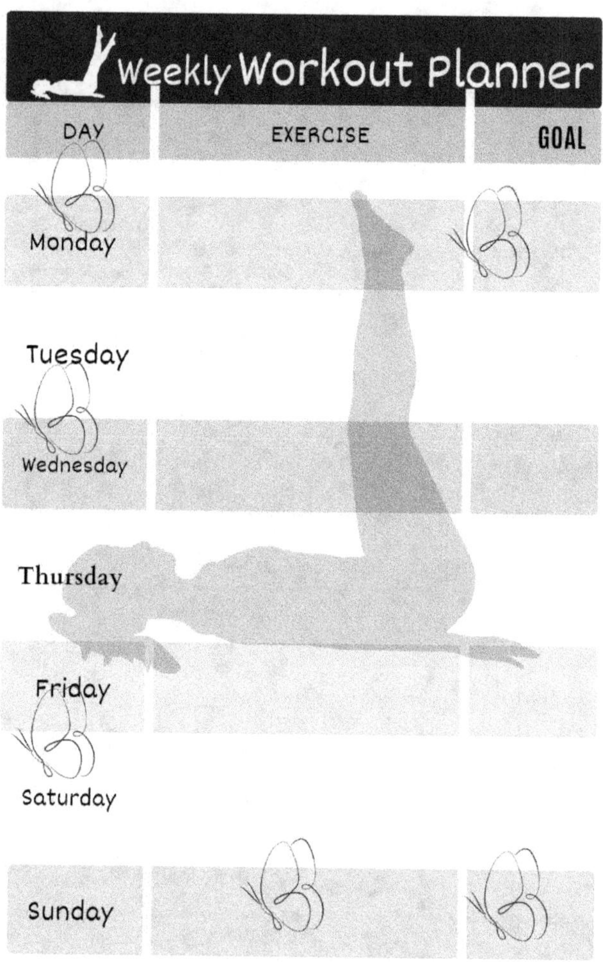

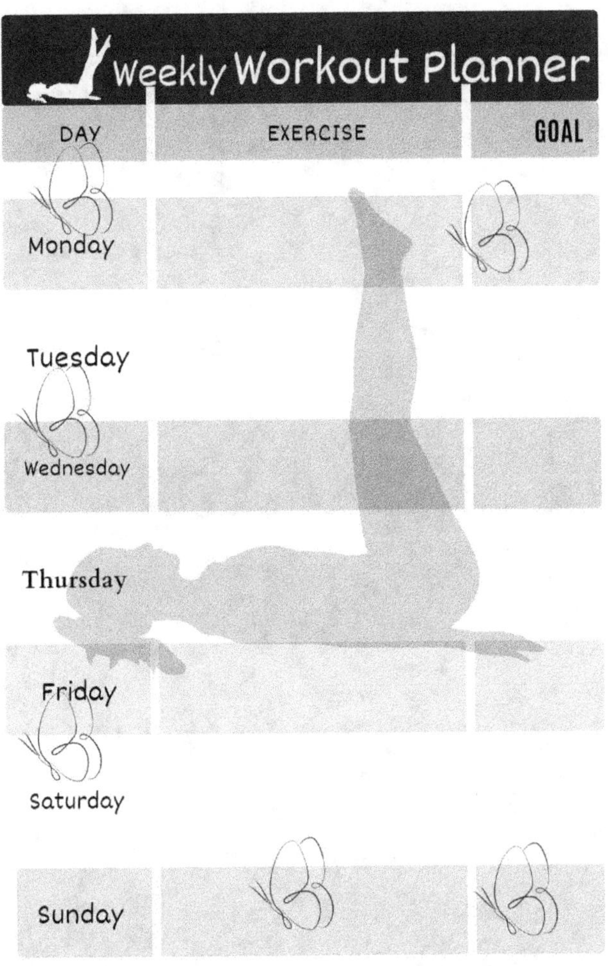
Weekly Workout Planner
DAY
EXERCISE
GOAL
Monday
Tuesday
Wednesday
Thursday
Friday
Saturday
Sunday

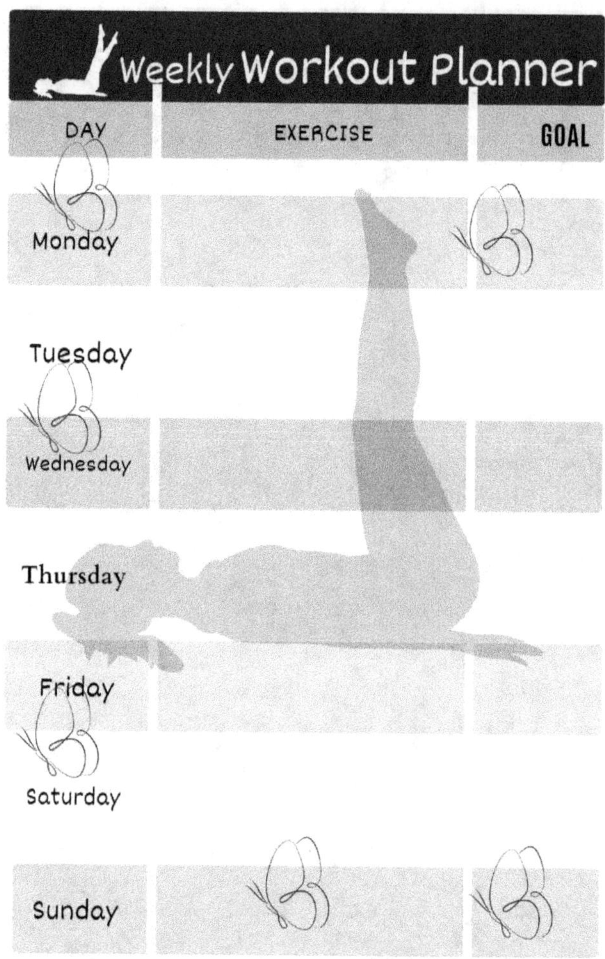

Weekly Workout Planner
DAY
EXERCISE
GOAL
Monday
Tuesday
Wednesday
Thursday
Friday
Saturday
Sunday

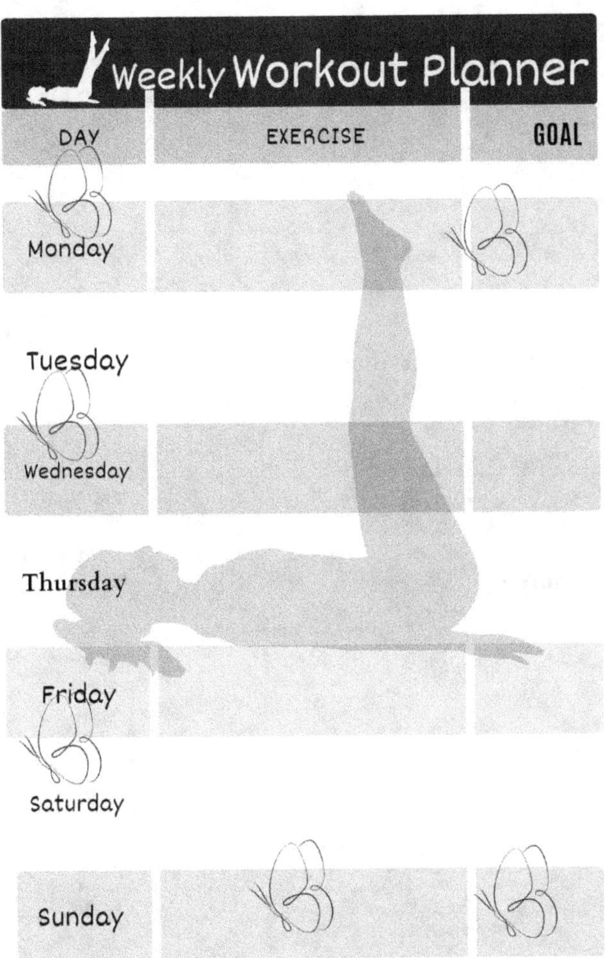

Weekly Workout Planner
DAY
EXERCISE
GOAL
Monday
Tuesday
Wednesday
Thursday
Friday
Saturday
Sunday

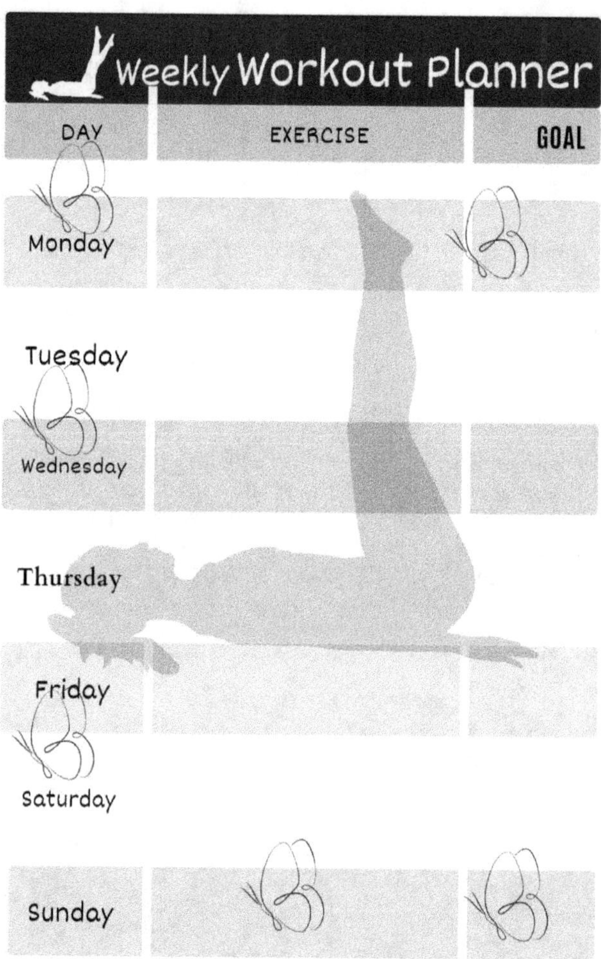
Weekly Workout Planner
DAY
EXERCISE
GOAL
Monday
Tuesday
Wednesday
Thursday
Friday
Saturday
Sunday

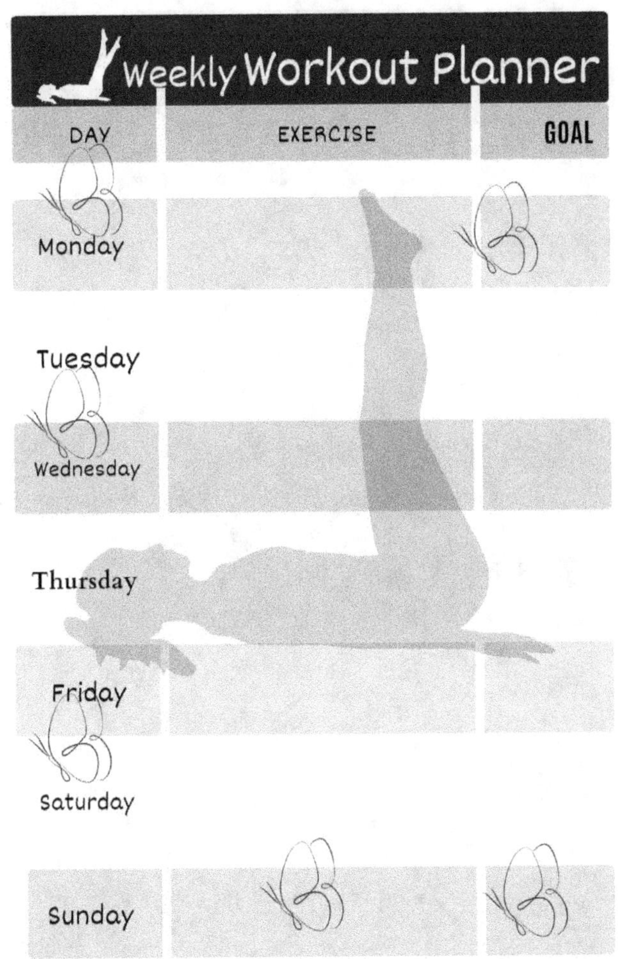

Weekly Workout Planner
DAY
EXERCISE
GOAL
Monday
Tuesday
Wednesday
Thursday
Friday
Saturday
Sunday

Weekly Workout Planner

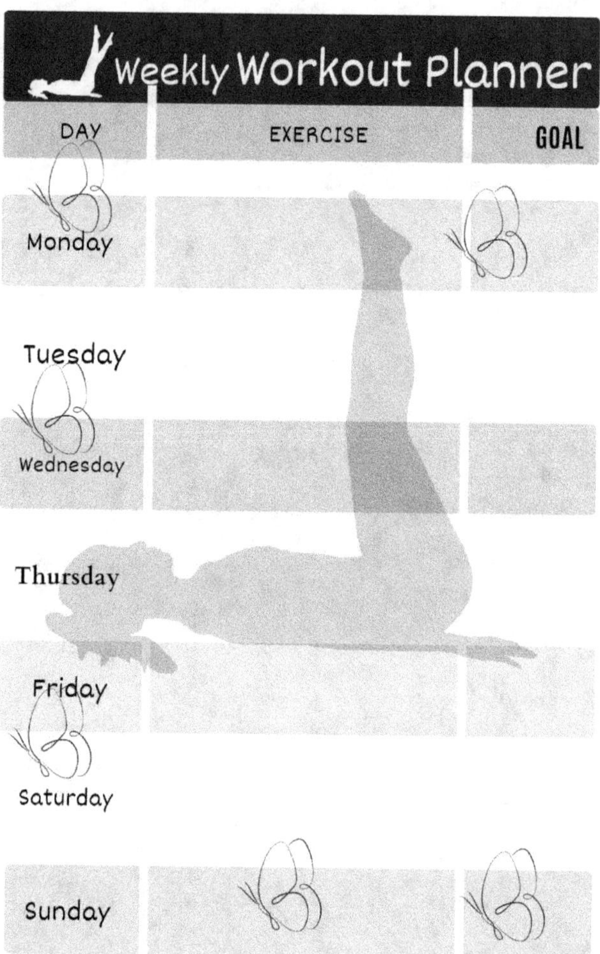

DAY	EXERCISE	GOAL
Monday		
Tuesday		
Wednesday		
Thursday		
Friday		
Saturday		
Sunday		

Weekly Workout Planner

DAY	EXERCISE	GOAL
Monday		
Tuesday		
Wednesday		
Thursday		
Friday		
Saturday		
Sunday		

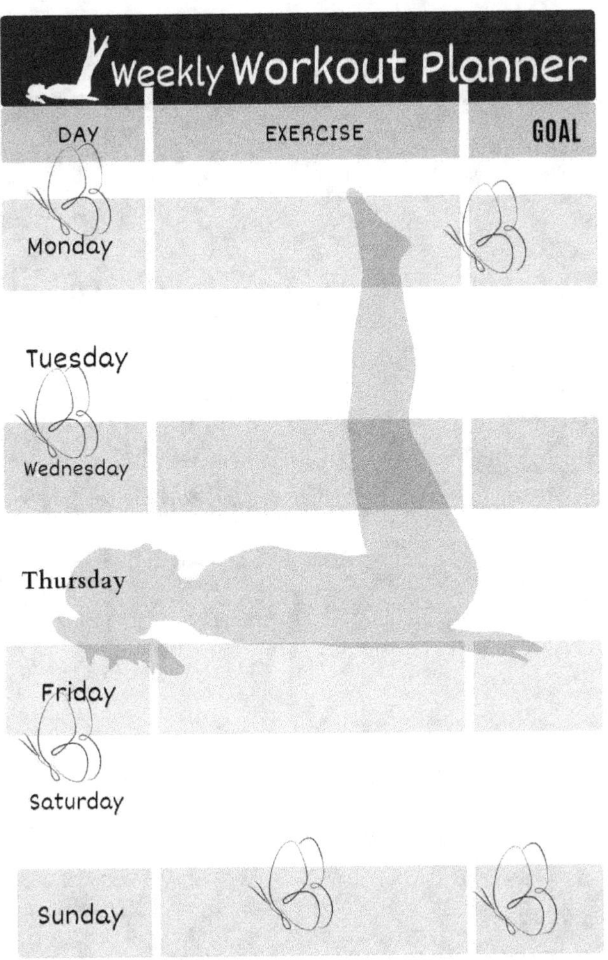

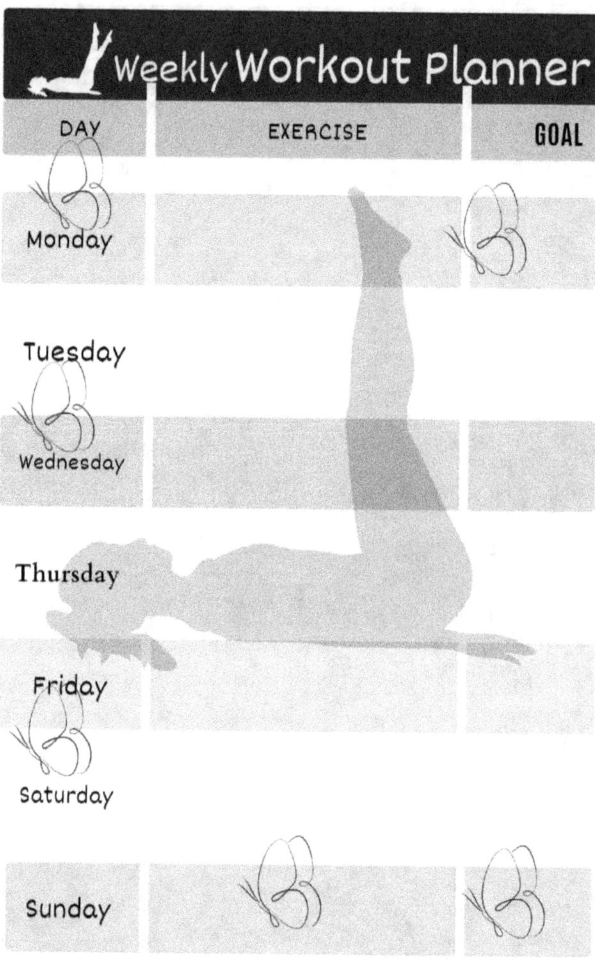
Weekly Workout Planner
DAY
EXERCISE
GOAL
Monday
Tuesday
Wednesday
Thursday
Friday
Saturday
Sunday

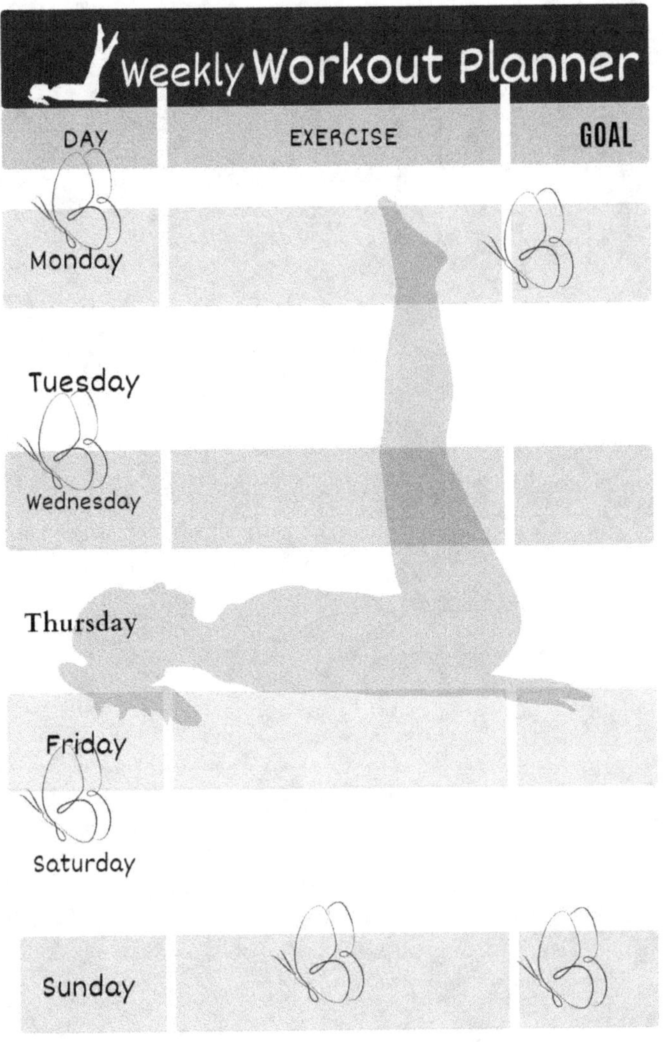

Weekly Workout Planner

DAY	EXERCISE	GOAL
Monday		
Tuesday		
Wednesday		
Thursday		
Friday		
Saturday		
Sunday